T0227147

Post-Polio Syndrome: Background, Management and Treatment

Editors

DARREN C. ROSENBERG
CRAIG ROVITO

PHYSICAL MEDICINE AND REHABILITATION CLINICS OF NORTH AMERICA

www.pmr.theclinics.com

Consulting Editor
SANTOS F. MARTINEZ

August 2021 • Volume 32 • Number 3

ELSEVIER

1600 John F. Kennedy Boulevard • Suite 1800 • Philadelphia, Pennsylvania, 19103-2899

http://www.theclinics.com

**PHYSICAL MEDICINE AND REHABILITATION CLINICS OF NORTH AMERICA Volume 32, Number 3
August 2021 ISSN 1047-9651, 978-0-323-76330-1**

Editor: Lauren Boyle
Developmental Editor: Diana Grace Ang

© **2021 Elsevier Inc. All rights reserved.**

This periodical and the individual contributions contained in it are protected under copyright by Elsevier, and the following terms and conditions apply to their use:

Photocopying
Single photocopies of single articles may be made for personal use as allowed by national copyright laws. Permission of the Publisher and payment of a fee is required for all other photocopying, including multiple or systematic copying, copying for advertising or promotional purposes, resale, and all forms of document delivery. Special rates are available for educational institutions that wish to make photocopies for non-profit educational classroom use. For information on how to seek permission visit www.elsevier.com/permissions or call: (+44) 1865 843830 (UK)/(+1) 215 239 3804 (USA).

Derivative Works
Subscribers may reproduce tables of contents or prepare lists of articles including abstracts for internal circulation within their institutions. Permission of the Publisher is required for resale or distribution outside the institution. Permission of the Publisher is required for all other derivative works, including compilations and translations (please consult www.elsevier.com/permissions).

Electronic Storage or Usage
Permission of the Publisher is required to store or use electronically any material contained in this periodical, including any article or part of an article (please consult www.elsevier.com/permissions). Except as outlined above, no part of this publication may be reproduced, stored in a retrieval system or transmitted in any form or by any means, electronic, mechanical, photocopying, recording or otherwise, without prior written permission of the Publisher.

Notice
No responsibility is assumed by the Publisher for any injury and/or damage to persons or property as a matter of products liability, negligence or otherwise, or from any use or operation of any methods, products, instructions or ideas contained in the material herein. Because of rapid advances in the medical sciences, in particular, independent verification of diagnoses and drug dosages should be made.

Although all advertising material is expected to conform to ethical (medical) standards, inclusion in this publication does not constitute a guarantee or endorsement of the quality or value of such product or of the claims made of it by its manufacturer.

Reprints. For copies of 100 or more of articles in this publication, please contact the Commercial Reprints Department, Elsevier Inc., 360 Park Avenue South, New York, NY 10010-1710. Tel.: 212-633-3874; Fax: 212-633-3820; E-mail: reprints@elsevier.com.

Physical Medicine and Rehabilitation Clinics of North America (ISSN 1047-9651) is published quarterly by Elsevier Inc., 360 Park Avenue South, New York, NY 10010-1710. Months of issue are February, May, August, and November. Business and Editorial Offices: 1600 John F. Kennedy Blvd., Suite 1800, Philadelphia, PA 19103-2899. Customer Service Office: 3251 Riverport Lane, Maryland Heights, MO 63043. Periodicals postage paid at New York, NY and additional mailing offices. Subscription price per year is $322.00 (US individuals), $879.00 (US institutions), $100.00 (US students), $366.00 (Canadian individuals), $923.00 (Canadian institutions), $100.00 (Canadian students), $463.00 (foreign individuals), $923.00 (foreign institutions), and $210.00 (foreign students). Foreign air speed delivery is included in all *Clinics* subscription prices. All prices are subject to change without notice. **POSTMASTER:** Send address changes to *Physical Medicine and Rehabilitation Clinics of North America*, Customer Service Office: Elsevier Health Sciences Division, Subscription Customer Service, 3251 Riverport Lane, Maryland Heights, MO 63043. **Customer Service: 1-800-654-2452 (US). From outside of the United States, call 314-447-8871. Fax: 314-447-8029. E-mail: JournalsCustomer Service-usa@elsevier.com (for print support); JournalsOnlineSupport-usa@elsevier.com (for online support).**

Physical Medicine and Rehabilitation Clinics of North America is indexed in *Excerpta Medica, MEDLINE/ PubMed (Index Medicus), Cinahl,* and *Cumulative Index to Nursing and Allied Health Literature.*

Contributors

CONSULTING EDITOR

SANTOS F. MARTINEZ, MD, MS
Diplomate, American Academy of Physical Medicine and Rehabilitation; Certificate of Added Qualification Sports Medicine, Assistant Professor, Department of Orthopaedics, Campbell Clinic Orthopaedics, University of Tennessee, Memphis, Tennessee

EDITORS

DARREN C. ROSENBERG, DO
Assistant Professor, Department of Physical Medicine and Rehabilitation, Harvard Medical School, Director, International Rehabilitation Center for Polio, Boston, Massachusetts

CRAIG ROVITO, MD
Instructor, Department of Physical Medicine and Rehabilitation, Traumatic Brain Injury Division, Spaulding Rehabilitation Hospital, Harvard Medical School, Boston, Massachusetts

AUTHORS

CAROL VANDENAKKER ALBANESE, MD
Professor, Department of Physical Medicine and Rehabilitation, UC Davis School of Medicine, Sacramento, California

KATE BRIZZI, MD
Instructor, Department of Neurology, Massachusetts General Hospital, Department of Medicine, Division of Palliative Care, Massachusetts General Hospital, Wang Ambulatory Care Center, Boston, Massachusetts

MARIA COLE, OTR, MHA
National Board for Certification in Occupational Therapy, Spaulding Outpatient Center Framingham, Framingham, Massachusetts

ANDREW DUBIN, MD, MS
Medical Director, UF Rehabilitation Hospital, Residency Program Director, Professor, Division of Physical Medicine and Rehabilitation, Department of Orthopedics and Rehabilitation Medicine, University of Florida, Gainesville, Florida

MIGUEL X. ESCALON, MD, MPH
Physical Medicine and Rehabilitation Vice Chair, Department of Rehabilitation and Human Performance, Icahn School of Medicine at Mount Sinai, New York, New York

BETH GRILL, PT, DPT
Board-Certified Clinical Specialist in Neurologic Physical Therapy, Spaulding Outpatient Center Framingham, Framingham, Massachusetts

WILLIAM IDE, MD
Department of Pediatric Rehabilitation, Kennedy Krieger Institute, Assistant Professor of Physical Medicine and Rehabilitation, Johns Hopkins School of Medicine, Baltimore, Maryland

EMILY KIVLEHAN, MD
Fellow, Pediatric Physical Medicine and Rehabilitation, Spaulding Rehabilitation Hospital, Mass General Brigham, Boston, Massachusetts

STEPHANIE T. MACHELL, PsyD
Independent Practice, Belmont, Massachusetts; Independent Practice, Framingham, Massachusetts

MICHELLE MELICOSTA, MD, MPH
Department of Pediatric Rehabilitation, Kennedy Krieger Institute, Assistant Professor of Pediatrics, Johns Hopkins School of Medicine, Baltimore, Maryland

JENNA RAHEB, PT, DPT, PCS
Physical Therapist and Owner, Raheb Physical Therapy, Adjunct Lecturer, Boston University, Physical Therapist, Spaulding Rehabilitation Hospital, Boston, Massachusetts

SHAILESH REDDY, MD
Neuromuscular Medicine Fellow, Department of Physical Medicine and Rehabilitation, UC Davis Health, Sacramento, California

JOHN Y. RHEE, MD, MPH
Department of Neurology, Massachusetts General Hospital, Brigham and Women's Hospital, Harvard Medical School, Wang Ambulatory Care Center, Boston, Massachusetts

ANGELA SAMAAN, DO
Physical Medicine and Rehabilitation Resident Physician, Department of Rehabilitation and Human Performance, Icahn School of Medicine at Mount Sinai, New York, New York

LAUREN T. SHAPIRO, MD, MPH
Assistant Professor of Clinical, Department of Physical Medicine and Rehabilitation, University of Miami Miller School of Medicine, Miami, Florida

ANDREW L. SHERMAN, MD, MS
Professor and Vice Chair of Education, Department of Physical Medicine and Rehabilitation, University of Miami Miller School of Medicine, Miami, Florida

MELISSA K. TROVATO, MD
Department of Pediatric Rehabilitation, Kennedy Krieger Institute, Assistant Professor of Physical Medicine and Rehabilitation, Johns Hopkins School of Medicine, Baltimore, Maryland

CLAUDIA A. WHEELER, DO, FAAPMR
Assistant Professor and Clinician Educator, Department of Neurosurgery, The Warren Alpert Medical School at Brown University, Medical Director, Adult Outpatient Rehabilitation, LPG Physiatry, Providence, Rhode Island

BRIAN D. WISHART, DO, MMS, FAAP
Attending Physician, Pediatric Physical Medicine and Rehabilitation, Spaulding Rehabilitation Hospital, Mass General Hospital for Children, Boston, Massachusetts

Contents

> Acute polio, once epidemic and a significant source of paralysis and disability, has been dramatically reduced through global vaccination programs. Although vaccination efforts have experienced a setback because of COVID-19, resulting in increased number of vaccine-associated and wild virus infections, polio eradication is still a realistic goal that will result in significant cost savings. The secondary health issues related to aging with the residual effects of polio, including postpolio syndrome, will persist for many years posteradication. Continued education of medical professionals is essential to ensure provision of the necessary care to this population.

> Acute flaccid myelitis (AFM) is an incompletely understood neurologic disorder occurring in epidemic fashion causing weakness ranging from mild paresis to devastating paralysis in children and some adults. This article reviews the case definition of AFM as well as its epidemiology and association with enteroviral infection. The clinical presentation, diagnostic investigation with particular attention to electrodiagnostics, acute management, and surgical options are described. Clinical outcomes and considerations for acute and long-term rehabilitation management are discussed extensively based on review of current literature, highlighting avenues for further study.

> Fatigue, a common complaint in individuals with postpolio syndrome (PPS), is defined as an overwhelming sustained feeling of exhaustion and diminished capacity for physical and mental work. A comprehensive medical work-up is needed to rule out all other causes of fatigue. A sleep study should be considered for individuals with PPS who complain of fatigue. Self-reported outcome measures, such as the Fatigue Severity Scale, are reliable and valid tools to measure fatigue in this population. Fatigue management consists of individualized treatment of underlying

medical conditions, energy conservation, pacing techniques, and lifestyle modifications.

The goals of bracing in polio and postpolio are to optimize joint position and support weak muscles with the goal of reducing falls, reducing deformities, and optimizing energy conservation. Orthoses are primarily used in the lower extremities to optimize gait. Less frequently, upper extremity orthoses are required. Polio survivors are at increased risk of falls and injuries. Appropriate bracing and compliance with the prescribed device can prevent falls and injuries. The best orthotic results are often achieved with patients who have significant deficits but walk regularly, are well motivated, and are willing to adapt their gait for orthotic use.

Acute poliomyelitis is now extremely rare in the United States. Worldwide there are still sporadic outbreaks, which are typically treated with acute inoculation programs. Although polio has effectively been eradicated, the full scope of the disease and its myriad manifestations both in the acute phase and in the postpolio syndrome phase, remain areas of fertile research, debate, and stimulating topics.

Postpolio syndrome (PPS) is a sequela with symptoms that often occur in patients who previously survived poliomyelitis. Pain is a characteristic feature of PPS. Although poliomyelitis is no longer commonly seen in the western world, there is a significant portion of patients living with PPS. Recognizing the signs of PPS is integral in developing treatment plans. Conservative management is routinely considered first-line therapy; however, alternate treatments, pharmacologic and minimally invasive, are used in more refractory cases. Approaching patients living with pain and PPS requires a holistic approach and an understanding of the efficacy of available treatment modalities.

Scoliosis has a very high prevalence among patients with neuromuscular disease involving the thoracic spine and truncal muscles. Physical examination and radiographs are used to screen for presence of scoliosis and monitor progression. Management includes therapy participation, optimizing equipment and orthotic use, and possible surgical intervention. Unlike idiopathic adolescent scoliosis, curves tend to progress despite orthotic use compliance. Associated pelvic obliquity creates risk for pressure sores and pain. As such, education of caregivers is a key point of optimizing management.

Stephanie T. Machell

Since the 1940s, the importance of addressing polio survivors' psychological issues along with their physical needs has been known. The clinical literature and polio survivors' narratives indicate positive responses to both psychotherapy and psychologically informed medical care for issues connected with acute polio and rehabilitation experiences as well as postpolio syndrome. Yet, barriers in the form of stigma and lack of awareness and resources prevent most from accessing such care. This article addresses the provision of polio-informed psychological treatment as well as ways of creating a culture that supports mental health within medical settings.

John Y. Rhee and Kate Brizzi

Palliative care is a team-based approach focusing on relief of physical, psychosocial, and existential distress and communication about serious illness. Patients with poliomyelitis and postpolio syndrome are at risk for contractures and can benefit from involvement of physical and occupational therapy. Hypersialorrhea can be treated with anticholinergic medications, botox, or radiation. Patients with dyspnea may require noninvasive positive pressure ventilation ± opioids or benzodiazepines. Constipation is often due to autonomic dysfunction and decreased mobility. There is a higher burden of anxiety. Early conversations about patients' goals and values as it relates to their health may help frame future decision-making.

Jenna Raheb

When providing health care services, clinicians should provide patient-centered and family-centered care. When providing care for medically complex patients, it is important to think about how health care teams are working together to care for patients. Health care providers need to think about how they can guide their patients to become more independent, have an improved quality of life, and have improved access to their homes and community environments when possible. Clinicians need to recognize the importance of caregivers and the burdens that are put on caregivers. Clinicians should provide support to caregivers whenever possible.

Lauren T. Shapiro and Andrew L. Sherman

Survivors of poliomyelitis may experience long-term sequelae that put them at increased risk for injury, pain, cardiovascular deconditioning, and functional decline. Osteoporotic fractures and entrapment neuropathies, in particular, may result in greater impairments in one's mobility and ability to perform activities of daily living. Dysphagia may necessitate the use of compensatory swallow strategies to minimize aspiration risk. Comorbid conditions, including hypertension, dyslipidemia, obesity, and stroke, are also very prevalent in this population. Risk factor modification, including diet, exercise, and medication compliance, is essential to achieve optimal health and function among survivors of poliomyelitis.

PHYSICAL MEDICINE AND REHABILITATION CLINICS OF NORTH AMERICA

SERIES OF RELATED INTEREST

Orthopedic Clinics
https://www.orthopedic.theclinics.com/
Neurologic Clinics
https://www.neurologic.theclinics.com/
Clinics in Sports Medicine
https://www.sportsmed.theclinics.com/

VISIT THE CLINICS ONLINE!
Access your subscription at:
www.theclinics.com

PHYSICAL MEDICINE AND REHABILITATION
CLINICS OF NORTH AMERICA

FORTHCOMING ISSUES

November 2021
Non-Spine Ablation Procedures
Santos F. Martinez, Editor

February 2022
Cycling
Angela Cortez and Dana Kotler, Editors

May 2022
Comprehensive Evidence Analysis for
Interventional Procedures Used to Treat
Chronic Pain
Alaa S. Abd-Elsayed, Editor

RECENT ISSUES

May 2021
Telerehabilitation
David X. Cifu and Blessen C. Eapen, Editors

February 2021
Dance Medicine
Kathleen L. Davenport, Editor

November 2020
Integrative Medicine and Rehabilitation
David X. Cifu and Blessen C. Eapen, Editors

SERIES OF RELATED INTEREST

Orthopedic Clinics
https://www.orthopedic.theclinics.com/

Neurologic Clinics
https://www.neurologic.theclinics.com/

Clinics in Sports Medicine
https://www.sportsmed.theclinics.com/

VISIT THE CLINICS ONLINE!
Access your subscription at:
www.theclinics.com

Foreword

We have nothing to fear except fear itself

—Franklin D. Roosevelt (1933)

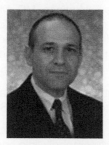

Santos F. Martinez, MD, MS
Consulting Editor

With challenges, opportunities and innovative strategies arise. Such was the case of Infantile Paralysis, which contributed a significant chapter to our field of Physical Medicine and Rehabilitation. National and international efforts took place to address this devastating condition; however, it was not until decades later that Poliomyelitis was eradicated from 99% of the globe. It was none other than Franklin D. Roosevelt who further brought national attention to this condition when he contracted the disease in the 1920s.

It was in the small unassuming town of Warm Springs, Georgia where a specialty hospital was developed to address this disease under Roosevelt's guidance and influence. The location was strategic from the perspective that there were naturally heated springs, which eventually were channeled to outdoor and subsequently indoor therapeutic pools. This was a special facility offering on-campus surgical, medical, orthotic, and allied health efforts. There was also a special spirit that engulfed not only the facility but also surrounding communities, which provided employees who learned skills that would be passed down for several generations as the Rehabilitation Hospital would later make transitions in treating other non-Polio conditions. These families were focused on potential rather than on disability. Despite significant physical impairments, these patients eventually became very active and productive in society, never asking for special accommodations or treatment. They just wanted the opportunity to experience the American dream, and that they did. This was exemplified by Franklin Roosevelt himself, who despite limitations became president for an unprecedented four terms extending from the Great Depression through World War 2. Despite his role in world affairs, he never forgot Warm Springs and eventually returned to live his remaining years at his "Little White House." This also was my first exposure to post-Polio patients and rehabilitation in general as a college extern at Warm Springs in 1977 and was the impetus that determined my career path. I hope this article gives us all reflection on what can be done rather than focusing on limitations. We have a lot to learn from our history and patients.

Phys Med Rehabil Clin N Am 32 (2021) xi–xii
https://doi.org/10.1016/j.pmr.2021.05.002
1047-9651/21/© 2021 Published by Elsevier Inc.

There are residual effects of Polio that we still see in the office from time to time. I hope this issue will help guide those clinicians who travel this journey with the Polio population through their various stages in life. I dedicate this effort to Dr James B. Knowles, who was a great clinician and mentor for the Roosevelt Warm Springs Rehabilitation family for several decades.

Santos F. Martinez, MD, MS
DiDepartment of Orthopaedics
Campbell Clinic Orthopaedics
University of Tennessee
Memphis, TN, USA

1400 South Germantown Road
Germantown, TN 38138, USA

E-mail address:
smartinez@campbellclinic.com

Preface

Pandemics Shaping our World

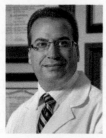 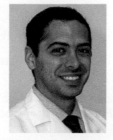

Darren C. Rosenberg, DO   Craig Rovito, MD
Editors

Afraid to leave the safety of my home and concerned about facing the invisible opponent that has been tormenting our community. Would someone in my family be ravaged by this virus that left so many neighbors with respiratory failure? Waiting for a cure, a magic antidote to the fear and suffering that has embraced not only our local community but also the world.

At the start of this project, most members of my generation would not have experienced this desperation. Polio was a distant memory to most and nearly absent from our medical school curriculum. I have heard these stories from numerous Polio survivors concerned about the late effects of this virus and the potential of possibly developing Postpolio Syndrome. Why study a virus that has been eradicated from the world except for a few war-torn countries?

The first cases began to be reported out of Wuhan, China. A highly contagious, deadly respiratory virus that seemed to appear out of the blue. My generation was presently being threatened by a deadly pandemic, COVID-19. Life has changed for all of us, and even mundane tasks became potentially life threatening.

A new appreciation of what Polio survivors lived through was thrust upon the world. Polio survivors continue to suffer from the late effects of their initial infection over a half century ago. The rich history that Polio survivors share with their practitioners cannot be forgotten, and this issue is necessary to update practitioners on the care of these patients. We now have seen firsthand how a pandemic affects the world population,

Phys Med Rehabil Clin N Am 32 (2021) xiii–xiv
https://doi.org/10.1016/j.pmr.2021.05.001
1047-9651/21/© 2021 Elsevier Inc. All rights reserved.

and we must listen to Polio survivors' stories and continue to provide them the best care available.

Darren C. Rosenberg, DO
Department of Physical Medicine and Rehabilitation
Harvard Medical School
Boston, MA, USA

International Rehabilitation Center for Polio
570 Worcester Road
Framingham, MA 01702, USA

Craig Rovito, MD
Department of Physical Medicine & Rehabilitation
Spaulding Rehabilitation Hospital/Harvard Medical School
300 First Avenue
Charlestown, MA 02129, USA

E-mail addresses:
drosenberg@partners.org (D.C. Rosenberg)
crovito@partners.org (C. Rovito)

The Current State
Epidemiology and Working Toward Eradication

Carol Vandenakker Albanese, MD[a],*, Shailesh Reddy, MD[b]

KEYWORDS

- Polio • Poliomyelitis • Postpolio syndrome • Polio sequelae
- Postpoliomyelitis syndrome

KEY POINTS

- Acute polio infections have been dramatically reduced through global vaccination programs.
- The World Health Organization has designated five of the six world regions as polio-free, reporting no recent cases of wild polio virus infection.
- Vaccination efforts have experienced a setback because of COVID-19, resulting in increased number of reported infections caused by wild virus in Afghanistan and Pakistan, the only countries with continued endemic polio virus, in 2020.
- Postpolio syndrome will continue for many years after eradication of polio has been achieved as survivors of acute polio age with residual weakness.

ACUTE POLIOMYELITIS
Polio Virus

Polio, or poliomyelitis, is the clinical presentation of infection with the poliovirus. The poliovirus is a member of the *Enterovirus* genus, Picornaviridae family. In the wild there are three serotypes: poliovirus 1, 2, and 3.[1] The virus is transmitted via excretion in feces and pharyngeal secretions with spread occurring in either oral-fecal or oral-oral manner. It then replicates in the gastrointestinal tract and can cause viremia and cross the blood-brain barrier.[2] Maximum virus excretion begins a few days before clinical symptoms and continues through the first week. The virus has a predilection for the anterior horn cells thus destroying motor neurons resulting in flaccid paralysis. It can also affect posterior horn cells, motor neurons of the thalamus, and hypothalamus.[3] Although paralysis is the most widely thought of presentation of disease, most cases are subclinical resulting in mild flulike illness. It is estimated that 1% to 5% of cases cause "nonparalytic aseptic meningitis" and less than 1% result in permanent paralysis.[4,5] Of the three serotypes, type 1 is most likely to cause paralysis, accounting for about 80% of cases.[6]

[a] Department of Physical Medicine and Rehabilitation, UC Davis School of Medicine, 4860 Y Street, Suite 3850, Sacramento, CA 95817, USA; [b] Department of Physical Medicine and Rehabilitation, UC Davis Health, 4860 Y Street, Suite 3850, Sacramento, CA 95817, USA
* Corresponding author.
E-mail address: cvalbanese@ucdavis.edu

Phys Med Rehabil Clin N Am 32 (2021) 467–476
https://doi.org/10.1016/j.pmr.2021.02.003
1047-9651/21/© 2021 Elsevier Inc. All rights reserved.

Acute Polio Infection

Clinically, patients present with a viral prodrome that may include any of the following: fever, headaches, neck stiffness, myalgias, fatigue, nausea, pharyngitis. The mild form of the disease usually subsides within a week. If the virus invades the central nervous system, severe muscle spasms and myalgias occur, which may be followed by asymmetrical flaccid paralysis, with sensory sparing. Muscle weakness is most profound during the acute stage of illness.

In the recovery stage, the paralysis may improve. Initial recovery is primarily through motor units recovering function. Secondary improvement occurs via axonal collateral sprouting, as residual motor units reinnervate adjacent denervated muscle fibers, resulting in enlarged or giant motor units. The recovery stage can last up to 2 years.[7]

Management of Acute Polio

Treatment during the acute and recovery stages is primarily supportive given that there are no antiviral medications approved for polio. Initially, management may include treatment of fever, prevention of respiratory infections and skin breakdown, and ventilatory support if respiratory muscles are affected. The paralyzed limbs are often splinted. Sister Elizabeth Kenny, an Australian nurse, introduced the notion of using hot packs to relieve muscle spasms. She also discouraged prolonged immobilization of the affected limbs.[3] Contracture prevention is an important part of management. During recovery, more intensive therapy is introduced with the tenets of nonfatiguing exercise and gradual progression of mobility and activities of daily living training. Orthotics and assistive devices are commonly used to support and protect weak muscles and joints. Surgical intervention may be used to reduce limb length discrepancy, restore useful function through tendon and muscle transfers, or prevention of deformity through tendon lengthening or joint fusion. More severely involved survivors may be wheelchair dependent or require ongoing ventilator assistance. A significant number of polio survivors have lived their entire lives dependent on the iron lung.

Differential Diagnosis

Other enteroviruses (enterovirus E71/D68, coxsackievirus A), West Nile virus, herpes zoster virus, Japanese encephalitis, and rabies can all cause similar presentations to acute poliomyelitis with flaccid paralysis.[8,9] Other potential causes of acute paralysis must also be considered including: acute inflammatory demyelinating polyradiculopathy, spinal cord infarction, myasthenia gravis, or rhabdomyolysis. Diagnostic tests used include: blood work, cerebrospinal fluid (CSF) analysis, stool tests, evaluation of respiratory function, electrodiagnostic studies, and central neuraxis MRI.

Prognosis

The extent and severity of paralytic polio symptoms is highly variable. Clinically, cases were identified as encephalitic, bulbar, spinal, or bulbospinal. In the early epidemics and in areas of the world with limited medical care, encephalitic and bulbar cases have a high mortality rate. The invention of the iron lung in 1928 with subsequent mass distribution at low cost significantly reduced the mortality rate.[5,10] Resultant paralysis varies from apparent full recovery (with reduced number of motor units in functional muscles) to localized single limb weakness, patchy weakness, or complete tetraplegia. Bulbar involvement often results in cranial nerve deficits, dysphagia, and respiratory problems.

Epidemiology

Polio did not start as an epidemic disease. One of the first known historical references goes back to a stone plaque, the Stele of Ruma, from ancient Egypt that dates back to the thirteenth century BC on which a priest with an atrophied limb and crutch is depicted. There were sporadic descriptions of acute febrile illness with paralysis, but few cases reported in the medical literature.[11]

In the late nineteenth century, reports of more widespread outbreaks in the United States and European countries started to appear.[12] By 1913, polio had been reported in every state with the first major US epidemic occurring in New York City in 1916.[13] Epidemics occurred regularly throughout the 1920s to 1950s, but were limited to Europe, United States, and Canada. The most prominent theory as to why the epidemics were localized to the western world is that with the development of improved sanitation, transmission of enteric infections was delayed until infants were older than 12 months, when the number of passive infant antibodies were reduced. Before the epidemic times, polio is thought to have been so common in the environment that infants were infected early in life when they had antibodies from their mothers, likely enough to prevent viremia and invasion of the central nervous system with subsequent paralysis.[11]

From the early 1900s through 1955 when the vaccine was introduced, the age distribution of those affected gradually increased, with the prevailing theory being because of reduction in circulation of the virus resulting in fewer early infections.[14] Longitudinal data from Sweden demonstrated that the rate of paralytic cases to number of infections does not increase with age, but the severity of the paralysis and fatality increases in the older population.[15] As public health improved in less developed countries, outbreaks of polio increased in those countries.[13]

Vaccine

The history of the development of the National Foundation for Infantile Paralysis, later to become the March of Dimes, which provided the funding and incentive that led to the race to develop a vaccine for polio, is a fascinating story.[16]

Albert Sabin and Jonas Salk were the primary scientists involved in vaccine development. The Salk vaccine, an inactivated polio vaccine (IPV) that is injected intramuscularly, was announced on April 12, 1955. The Sabin vaccine, the oral polio vaccine (OPV) that uses attenuated virus, became available in 1961. After release of the Sabin vaccine, the benefits of increased immunogenicity in the community through spread of the weakened live virus from those immunized (children) to others (adults and unvaccinated children) and easier administration led to predominate use of the OPV.

There is risk of vaccine-related polio infection caused by the OPV. The vaccine-induced polio (VAPP) occurs in an estimated 1 to 2 cases per million primary immunizations among vaccines and their close contacts. When entire families are vaccinated, almost all cases occur in vaccines; when immunization was only given to children, cases occurred in about equal numbers among close contacts. About 20% of vaccine-associated infection was reported in children with immunodeficiency. The risk of VAPP varies by serotype with normal vaccines at highest risk from type 3 virus, immunodeficient recipients, and contacts at highest risk from type 2. As of 1997, the US immunization recommendation was changed to one dose of IPV before OPV. In 2000 the recommendation was to use IPV exclusively, eliminating cases of VAPP in the United States.[17]

Polio Eradication

As the vaccines were disseminated through the United States, the incidence of polio fell dramatically. The last cases caused by indigenous wild poliovirus occurred in

1972. Subsequent cases in the United States were either vaccine-associated or imported.[18] In 1979 the United States was declared polio-free, although vaccine associated cases continued into the 1990s.

The eradication of wild poliovirus in the United States was not initially expected, but with the success of the vaccination programs in the developed countries, eradication of wild polio in other regions became plausible. Success in Cuba and Brazil led the Pan American Health Organization to start an aggressive campaign to eradicate the virus in the Americas. The program included routine pediatric immunizations supplemented by mass immunization days and mop-up in outbreak areas, providing at least three doses of the OPV to about 80% of children by the age of 1 year.[19]

With the success of the eradication campaign in the Americas, in 1988 the World Health Assembly established the Global Polio Eradication Initiative (GPEI) with a goal for global eradication of the wild polio virus.[20] The GPEI is a public-private partnership, which includes the World Health Organization (WHO), the United Nations Children's Fund, the US Centers for Disease Control and Prevention, the Bill and Melinda Gates Foundation, and Rotary International.[21] The initiative has been successful, but an early goal of global eradication by the year 2000 was not achieved. Worldwide cases were reduced from approximately 50,000 in 1980 to less than 1000 in 2001. By 2001, the number of countries with endemic wild polio had been reduced from more than 100 to less than 10. The original goal of eradication by the year 2000 has been delayed because of several factors.

Factors leading to delay in polio eradication:

- Interruption of transmission of the virus is more difficult in tropical climates that lack seasonal variation in case numbers.[22]
- Administration of OPV to children concurrently infected with other enteroviruses is less effective.
- Conversion rates with use of trivalent OPV (protective against serotypes 1, 2, and 3) is lower than with monovalent.
- Emergence of vaccine-derived polio virus (cVDPV), which occurs when the attenuated virus in the oral vaccine regains virulence circulating in an underimmunized population,[23] identified in 2000.
- cVDPV outbreaks occur when less than 50% of children receive the recommended three doses of OPV during immunization programs.

The WHO certifies individual countries and world regions (Africa, Americas, Eastern Mediterranean, Europe, South-East Asia, and Western Pacific) as polio-free. To be certified, a region needs to: record no wild polio case for at least 3 years, have a reliable surveillance system, and prove its capacity to detect and respond to imported cases of polio.[21]

With the decline in incidences of poliomyelitis caused by the wild virus, the cases of paralysis from vaccine-associated paralytic polio and vaccine-derived polio virus became more frequent than those related to wild virus. More than 90% of the vaccine-derived cases were caused by type 2, the wild type of which had been certified as globally eradicated in 2015. In 2016, the GPEI and the WHO switched from the trivalent OPV to a bivalent OPV protective against serotypes 1 and 3. The GPEI also recommended that at least one dose of IPV precede routine immunization with OPV. In October 2019, eradication of WPV type 3, last detected in 2012, was certified.[23]

In 2017, the virus was endemic in three countries: Nigeria, Afghanistan, and Pakistan. Nigeria has had no evidence of wild polio virus since September of 2016, and on August 25, 2020, Africa was officially certified as free of the wild polio virus.[18]

The most recent vaccination data from 2018 estimate global coverage of recommended routine immunization with three doses of poliovirus vaccine among infants younger than age 1 as 89%. Those receiving the recommended one full or two fractional doses of IPV is 72%.[24]

Current Status

At this time, two of the three wild polio serotypes (type 2 and 3) have been eradicated. Wild polio virus serotype 1 remains persistent only in Afghanistan and Pakistan.

In 2019, Afghanistan and Pakistan reported a significant increase in the number of endemic polio infections, 176 cases.[21] Between January 1, 2020, and August 12, 2020, 85 WPV1 cases were reported, compared with 64 year to date in 2019. Both countries continue to face problems with mobile populations, vaccine refusal, and polio campaign fatigue.[25] Continued political unrest in Afghanistan has led to temporary restrictions and banning of the vaccination effort.

In addition, since the change to bivalent OPV in 2016, type 2 cVDPV outbreaks have increased in number and countries reporting. To date in 2020, 210 cVDPV cases have been reported compared with 69 in 2019. Since 2018, cVDPV outbreaks have affected four of the six WHO world regions (Africa, Eastern Mediterranean, South-East Asia, and Western Pacific). Outbreaks are treated with monovalent OPV2 vaccines. A new genetically stabilized novel OPV2 (nOPV2) with lower risk of conversion to virulent form has been developed for distribution later this year.[26]

Impact of COVID-19

In March 2020, GPEI committed its laboratory and surveillance network and workers to support preparedness and response to the COVID-19 pandemic. This included postponing outbreak response mass immunization campaigns until June and preventive mass immunization campaigns until the second half of 2020. Surveillance continued, although with disruptions. In July 2020 outbreak responses resumed but preventative campaigns are still on hold.[27]

Pakistan and Afghanistan are fighting increased numbers of wild virus cases and outbreaks of vaccine-related polio virus infections. It is essential that community engagement and trust be re-established and the management and provision of health services improved to reach the chronically missed children.[23]

Endgame

It is estimated that since it was started, the GPEI has prevented 18 million cases of paralysis and 1.5 million childhood deaths. Eradication of polio will translate into significant economic savings, estimated at $40 to $50 billion US dollars (in vaccination costs and in relation to impact of the disease). More importantly, it will mean elimination of lifelong paralysis caused by the polio virus, postpolio syndrome, and its subsequent impact on health and society.

POSTPOLIO SYNDROME
History

The diagnosis of postpolio syndrome gained recognition in the 1970s and 1980s when several acute polio survivors started to present with new symptoms of increased weakness and fatigue.[28] Although the sequelae of the polio epidemics was not felt until this time period, the first reported cases of postpolio syndrome can be traced back to 1875, when French neurologist Jean Martin-Charcot described three young men, who all had polio as infants, and who developed new-onset weakness and atrophy during their adult years.[29] Early reports in the medical literature used several different terms to describe the symptoms that polio survivors were experiencing, including "postpolio muscular atrophy," "the late effects of polio," "postpolio sequelae," and "postpolio syndrome."

In 1984, a scientific conference for clinicians and researchers was held at the Roosevelt Warm Springs Institute for Rehabilitation to define postpolio syndrome. The conference attracted the attention of the news media, many of whom attended the final day. Reports sparked fear of polio virus reactivation and another polio epidemic. The interest generated by this false narrative led to increased research and the establishment of multiple support groups and 96 specialty clinics in response to deal with what had yet to be recognized as postpolio syndrome. A subsequent conference at Warm Springs Institute in 1986 helped to further legitimize postpolio syndrome as a greater number of researchers from seven countries presented evidence that postpolio syndrome was a distinct clinical entity.[28]

Despite the increasing number of cases of polio survivors presenting with new weakness and expanding medical literature on the subject, postpolio syndrome was not fully legitimized as a diagnosis until 1994. A conference hosted by the National Institutes of Health and the New York Academy of Sciences brought together prominent polio researchers from across the globe[29] to present and discuss current understanding. Today, postpolio syndrome is a well-recognized entity; however, much remains unknown about pathophysiology and the true prevalence.

Current Prevalence

The true prevalence of postpolio syndrome remains unclear. Because no national database of polio survivors exists, it is difficult to ascertain accurate disease statistics. In 2010, the March of Dimes estimated that there were between 10 and 20 million polio survivors globally. More recently in 2016, Groce and colleagues[30] narrowed that estimate to 15 to 20 million with an estimated 573,000 survivors in the United States. Because of the nature of the disease, many cases of mild polio may be missed in the estimates. Given that the estimate of polio survivors is fundamentally inaccurate, it follows that the number of survivors who develop postpolio syndrome shares the same inaccuracies.

Prevalence ranges for postpolio syndrome are generally broad and highly variable. One 1994 to 1995 survey estimated that the prevalence of postpolio syndrome ranged from 11% to 25%,[28] but Ramlow and colleagues[31] estimated that the prevalence of postpolio syndrome may be up to 78%. In 2005, Ragonese and colleagues[32] published an estimate of 20% to 100%. The reasons that the estimates vary so greatly include variation in populations studied, differing diagnostic criteria used for assessment, and variable study duration.

Pathogenesis

Although postpolio syndrome is now a well-recognized entity, pathophysiology is not completely understood. The most widely accepted theory was proposed by Weichers and Hubbell[33] in 1981. They hypothesized that the symptoms of new muscle weakness and fatigability are caused by distal degeneration of axon sprouts supplied by enlarged motor units that developed during the recovery of acute polio resulting in denervation of muscle fibers.[33] This theory has been supported by histologic studies that found isolated, angular, atrophic fibers on muscle biopsy of postpolio patients. This implies local denervation as opposed to entire muscle group atrophy indicative of the loss of entire motor units, such as in amyotrophic lateral sclerosis.[34] Although this hypothesis provides a general framework for the pathophysiology of postpolio muscle weakness it does not delineate factors that may contribute to the distal axonal sprout degeneration.

Other hypotheses have expanded on the explanation proposed by Weichers and Hubbell. The normal process of aging has been postulated to have a significant effect on the development of postpolio syndrome. The neuromuscular sequelae of normal aging include: a reduction in the total number of muscle fibers and motor units, sarcopenia, lean tissues loss, and decreased strength because of deconditioning. When these consequences are superimposed on the already limited number of motor neurons caused by polio infection it may contribute to progressive loss of strength and lead to development of symptoms consistent with postpolio syndrome.[34,35] Aging has also been shown to decrease levels of circulating growth hormone and insulin-like growth factor-1. These hormones have been linked with the development of axonal sprouting and muscle fiber hypertrophy; therefore, their absence may contribute to the degeneration of distal axonal sprouts. Although there seems to be significant rationale for the contribution of aging to the development of postpolio syndrome, studies have been conflicting in confirmation of aging as a risk factor.[36]

Overuse myopathy has also been theorized as a mechanism contributing to the development of postpolio syndrome. Some studies have described the finding of elevated creatine kinase in symptomatic patients directly correlated significantly with distance of ambulation, the implication being that increased activity contributes to the development of postpolio syndrome.[37] Peach[38] reported a case where clinical intervention of reduced activity resulted in symptom resolution and decline in serum creatine kinase.

Theories of poliovirus reactivation or persistence have been controversial. Studies have described the presence of poliovirus RNA in the CSF of patients with postpolio syndrome but additional studies did not confirm either viral fragments or poliovirus-specific immunoglobulin antibodies.[39] An immune or inflammatory response to these viral fragments has been postulated based on increased levels of proinflammatory cytokines in the CSF of postpolio patients leading to clinical trials of intravenous immunoglobulin treatment of postpolio syndrome.[40] Not all patients respond to treatment and further evaluation of responders and nonresponders has led to a hypothesis that the pathogenesis may vary.[41]

In summary, there is no consensus for the exact pathophysiology of postpolio syndrome. Wiechers and Hubbell proposed the most widely accepted hypothesis that seems to explain the development of the new muscle weakness reported in postpolio syndrome. Other explanations, such as factors associated with aging, overuse myopathy, and immunologic response, may contribute to pathophysiology. It is likely that not all patients have the same pathogenesis but rather a combination of etiologies that contribute to the symptoms of postpolio syndrome.

Diagnosis

A specific diagnostic test for postpolio syndrome does not exist; however, diagnostic criteria have been developed by a consensus of experts. These criteria have changed over the years. The guidelines that are the most widely accepted currently were published in 2000 by the March of Dimes (**Box 1**).[42] The most common complaint exhibited by patients is either fatigue or weakness. With an aging patient population these symptoms are experienced in a wide range of diagnoses spanning multiple organ systems.[36] For this reason, many tests may be necessary to arrive at the diagnosis of postpolio syndrome given it is a diagnosis of exclusion. MRI of the lumbar spine and electrodiagnostic studies can assess for spinal or peripheral nerve or muscle pathology. Laboratory work, such as complete blood count, complete metabolic panel, and

---

Box 1
March of Dimes criteria for postpoliomyelitis syndrome

Prior paralytic poliomyelitis with evidence of motor neuron loss, as confirmed by history of the acute paralytic illness, signs of residual weakness and atrophy of muscles on neurologic examination, and signs of denervation on electromyography.

A period of partial or complete functional recovery after acute paralytic poliomyelitis, followed by an interval (usually 15 years or more) of stable neurologic function.

Gradual or sudden onset of progressive and persistent new muscle weakness or abnormal muscle fatigability (decreased endurance), with or without generalized fatigue, muscle atrophy, or muscle and joint pain. Sudden onset may follow a period of inactivity, or trauma or surgery. Less commonly, symptoms attributed to postpolio syndrome include new problems with breathing or swallowing.

Symptoms persist for at least 1 year.

Exclusion of other neurologic, medical, and orthopedic problems as causes of symptoms.

---

thyroid studies, can assess contributing factors of anemia, electrolyte imbalance, and hypothyroidism. Pulmonary function testing and sleep studies may identify sleep apnea or hypoventilation with hypercarbia. These tests serve to exclude diagnoses other than postpolio syndrome as explanatory etiologies for presenting symptoms; they do not provide findings that are sensitive or specific to postpolio syndrome. Although identification of concurrent problems does not confirm diagnosis, medical management of identified contributing conditions can reduce the symptoms of postpolio syndrome.

SUMMARY

Eradication of acute poliovirus is still an achievable goal that despite recent setbacks because of Covid-19 should be attainable in the next decade. Despite decreasing numbers of acute polio infections, postpolio syndrome will remain a clinical problem for many survivors of paralytic polio as they age for years to come. Clinicians need to be educated and aware of the conditions associated with sequelae of polio to provide the needed medical care and rehabilitation interventions that this population requires.

DISCLOSURE

The authors have nothing to disclose.

REFERENCES

1. Brown B, Oberste MS, Maher K, et al. Complete genomic sequencing shows that polioviruses and members of human enterovirus species C are closely related in the noncapsid coding region. J Virol 2003;77(16):8973–84.
2. Bodian D. Emerging concept of poliomyelitis infection. Science 1955;122(3159): 105–8.
3. Mehndiratta MM, Mehndiratta P, Pande R. Poliomyelitis: historical facts, epidemiology, and current challenges in eradication. Neurohospitalist 2014;4(4):223–9.
4. Nathanson N, Martin JR. The epidemiology of poliomyelitis: enigmas surrounding its appearance, epidemicity, and disappearance. Am J Epidemiol 1979;110(6): 672–92.

5. Ochmann S. Polio. 2017. Available at: https://ourworldindata.org/polio. Accessed August 10, 2020.
6. Centers for Disease Control and Prevention. Poliomyelitis surveillance report, number 65. Atlanta (GA): Centers for Disease Control and Prevention; 1956.
7. Howard RS. Poliomyelitis and the postpolio syndrome. BMJ 2005;330(7503): 1314–8.
8. Helfferich J, Knoester M, Van Leer-Buter CC, et al. Acute flaccid myelitis and enterovirus D68: lessons from the past and present. Eur J Pediatr 2019;178(9): 1305–15.
9. Kawajiri S, Tani M, Noda K, et al. Segmental zoster paresis of limbs: report of three cases and review of literature. Neurologist 2007 Sep;13(5):313–7.
10. The Iron Lung and Other Equipment. Web site. Available at: https://amhistory.si.edu/polio/howpolio/ironlung.htm. Accessed August 10, 2020.
11. Nathanson N, Kew OM. From emergence to eradication: the epidemiology of poliomyelitis deconstructed. Am J Epidemiol 2010;172:1213–29.
12. Lavinder CH, Freeman AW, Frost WH. Epidemiologic studies of poliomyelitis in New York City and the Northeastern United States during the year 1916. Washington, DC: US GPO; 1918.
13. Paul JR. A History of poliomyelitis. New Haven (CT): Yale University Press; 1971.
14. Dauer CC. The changing age distribution of paralytic poliomyelitis. Ann N Y Acad Sci 1955;61(4):943–55.
15. Olin G. The epidemiologic pattern of poliomyelitis in Sweden from 1905 to 1950. In: Fishbein M, editor. Poliomyelitis: papers and discussions presented at the second international poliomyelitis conference. Philadelphia: J B Lippincott & Company; 1952. p. 367–75.
16. Oshinsky DM. Polio: an American story. New York: Oxford University Press; 2005.
17. Alexander LN, Seward JF, Santibanez TA, et al. Vaccine policy changes and epidemiology of poliomyelitis in the United States. JAMA 2004;292(14):1696–701.
18. Polio. Website. Available at: https://www.cdc.gov/polio/what-is-polio/index.htm. Accessed August 25, 2020.
19. Certification of poliomyelitis eradication—the Americas, 1994. MMWR Morb Mortal Wkly Rep 1994;43(39):720–2.
20. World Health Assembly. Polio eradication by the year 2000. Geneva (Switzerland): World Health Organization; 1988.
21. Poliomyelitis. Web site. 2019. Available at: https://www.who.int/news-room/fact-sheets/detail/poliomyelitis. Accessed August 10, 2020.
22. Patriarca PA, Wright PF, John TJ. Factors affecting the immunogenicity of oral poliovirus vaccine in developing countries: review. Rev Infect Dis 1991;13(5): 926–39.
23. Chard AN, Datta SD, Tallis G, et al. Progress toward polio eradication—worldwide, January 2018-March 2020. MMWR Morb Mortal Wkly Rep 2020;69(25): 784–9.
24. Martinez M, Shukla H, Ahmadzai M, et al. Progress toward poliomyelitis eradication—Afghanistan, January 2017–August 2018. MMWR Morb Mortal Wkly Rep 2018;67:833–7.
25. Patel JC, Diop OM, Gardner T, et al. Surveillance to track progress toward polio eradication—worldwide, 2017–2018. MMWR Morb Mortal Wkly Rep 2019;68: 312–8.
26. Greene SA, Ahmed J, Datta SD, et al. Progress toward polio eradication—worldwide, January 2017-March 2019. MMWR Morb Mortal Wkly Rep 2019;68(20): 458–62.

27. Roberts L. Polio vaccinators are back after pandemic pause. Science 2020; 369(6502):360.
28. Halstead L. A brief history of post polio syndrome in the United States. Arch Phys Med Rehabil 2011;92:1344–9.
29. Dalakas MC, Bertfield H, Kurland LT. The post polio syndrome: advances in the pathogenesis and treatment. Ann N Y Acad Sci 1995;753:1–412.
30. Groce NE, Banks LM, Stein MA. Surviving polio in a post polio world. Soc Sci Med 2014;107:171–8.
31. Ramlow J, Alexander M, LaPorte R, et al. Epidemiology of the post polio syndrome. Am J Epidemiol 1992;136:769–86.
32. Ragonese P, Fierro B, Salemi G, et al. Prevalence and risk factors of post-polio syndrome in a cohort of polio survivors. J Neurol Sci 2005;236:31–5.
33. Wiechers DO, Hubbell SL. Late changes in the motor unit after acute poliomyelitis. Muscle Nerve 1981;4:524–8.
34. Bickerstaffe A, van Dijk JP, Beelen A, et al. Loss of motor unit size and quadriceps strength over 10 years in post polio syndrome. Clin Neurophysiol 2014;125: 1255–60.
35. Gordon T, Hegedus J, Tam SL. Adaptive and maladaptive motor axonal sprouting in aging and motor neuron disease. Neurol Res 2004;26(2):174–85.
36. Lo J, Robinson L. Postpolio syndrome and the late effects of poliomyelitis. Part 1. Pathogenesis, biomechanical considerations, diagnosis, and investigations. Muscle Nerve 2018;58:751–9.
37. Trojan D, Cashman N. Post-poliomeylitis syndrome. Muscle Nerve 2005;31:6–19.
38. Peach PE. Overwork weakness with evidence of muscle damage in a patient with residual paralysis from polio. Arch Phys Med Rehabil 1990;71:248–50.
39. Cashman NR, Meselli R, Wollman RI, et al. Late denervation in patients with antecedent paralytic poliomyelitis. N Engl J Med 1987;317:7–12.
40. Gonzalez H, Khademi M, Borg K, et al. Intravenous immunoglobulin treatment of the post-polio syndrome: sustained effects on quality of life variables and cytokine expression after one-year follow-up. J Neuroinflammation 2012;9:167.
41. Östlund G, Broman L, Werhagen L, et al. Immunoglobulin treatment in post-polio syndrome: identification of responders and non-responders. J Rehabil Med 2015; 47(8):727–33.
42. March of Dimes. Post polio syndrome: identifying the best practices in diagnosis and care. White Plains (NY): March of dimes Birth Defects Foundation; 2001.

Acute Flaccid Myelitis

William Ide, MD[a,b], Michelle Melicosta, MD, MPH[a,c],
Melissa K. Trovato, MD[a,b],*

KEYWORDS

• Acute • Flaccid • Myelitis • Paralysis • Enterovirus • Polio-like • EV-D68

KEY POINTS

• Acute flaccid myelitis (AFM) is an emerging polio-like illness predominately affecting children with the potential to cause severe disability.

• Outbreaks have occurred in the United States every 2 years since 2012 with peaks in September, coinciding with peaks in enterovirus infections, although the exact pathogenesis is unclear.

• Clinical presentation is typically acute onset of asymmetric paralysis in one or more limbs with longitudinal hyperintensities largely affecting the spinal cord gray matter on MRI.

• There are various empiric treatments used during acute disease, but no definitive therapy has been proven to improve outcomes at this time.

• Comprehensive rehabilitation is key to address the impact of AFM upon multiple body systems, and ongoing surveillance is necessary to monitor long-term outcomes.

INTRODUCTION

Acute flaccid myelitis (AFM) is a polio-like illness primarily affecting previously healthy children, characterized by acute flaccid paralysis (AFP) of one or more limbs associated with injury to the spinal cord gray matter following a prodromal illness. In 2012, a case of AFP with anterior myelitis in a 29-year-old unvaccinated man with no travel history was reported to the California Department of Public Health (CDPH).[1] Between 2012 and 2014, the CDPH identified a total of 23 cases of AFP with myelitis in which epidemiologic and laboratory investigation did not identify poliovirus infection as a possible cause.[1] From August through October 2014, another cluster of 11 children presenting with acute limb weakness, with and without cranial nerve dysfunction, and radiologic findings of myelitis was reported in Aurora, Colorado.[2] In response, the term AFM was coined by the Centers for Disease Control and

[a] Department of Pediatric Rehabilitation, Kennedy Krieger Institute, 707 North Broadway, Ste. 232, Baltimore, MD 21205, USA; [b] Department of Physical Medicine & Rehabilitation, Johns Hopkins University School of Medicine; [c] Department of Pediatrics, Johns Hopkins University School of Medicine
* Corresponding author. Department of Pediatric Rehabilitation, Kennedy Krieger Institute, 707 North Broadway, Ste. 232, Baltimore, MD 21205.
E-mail address: trovato@kennedykrieger.org

Phys Med Rehabil Clin N Am 32 (2021) 477–491
https://doi.org/10.1016/j.pmr.2021.02.004
1047-9651/21/© 2021 Elsevier Inc. All rights reserved.

Prevention (CDC) to describe this recognized syndrome of AFP in which cord myelitis has been documented, typically via MRI visualization.[2,3] Since then, a national call for cases published by the CDC has identified seasonal waves of cases occurring in a biennial pattern in the United States, the most recent in 2018.[3,4] A strong association with non-polio enterovirus (NPEV) infection has been supported by epidemiologic evidence, although a viral pathogen is frequently not isolated in cases of AFM.[2,3,5,6]

Clinical presentations of AFM are variable and range from mild impairments to requirement for intensive care and invasive ventilatory support. Neurologic symptoms may be rapidly progressive following a febrile illness, typically respiratory, although AFM may arise following gastrointestinal or hand-foot-mouth disease symptoms.[4] Diagnosis may be confounded by difficulty in distinguishing AFM from neurologic disorders to include spinal cord ischemia, transverse myelitis, acute disseminated encephalomyelitis, and peripheral inflammatory myelopathies.[6,7] MRI of the spinal axis with and without contrast will reveal longitudinal lesions of the spinal cord gray matter with selective involvement of the anterior horns.[6,7]

Close monitoring and supportive care are central to the early management of AFM given the risk for precipitous respiratory deterioration and autonomic instability. Currently, no singular medical therapy has been endorsed by the CDC AFM Task Force on the basis of insufficient evidence.[8,9] Although high-quality clinical trials are lacking, several therapeutic strategies are commonly used in acute AFM, all without conclusive evidence of efficacy.[7,9] Comprehensive rehabilitation is beneficial to maximize function, and some patients may benefit from nerve transfer surgery.[10,11] As in other aspects of the disease, recovery in AFM is variable, and ongoing surveillance will be necessary to describe long-term outcomes and facilitate prognosis. Most patients regain some degree of function with persistence of motor deficits at 12- to 18-month follow-up.[12,13]

CASE DEFINITIONS

The September 26, 2014 call for national reporting issued via the CDC's Health Alert Network stipulated the following criteria to confirm AFM: (1) Acute onset of focal limb weakness AND predominant gray matter lesions on spinal MRI, (2) person 21 years of age or younger, and (3) occurring on or after August 1, 2014.[14] In June 2015, the Council of State and Territorial Epidemiologists (CSTE) adopted a standardized case definition for AFM that is used by the CDC.[15,16] This case definition removed the age restriction to include adults greater than 21 years of age, allowed for classification of cases as "confirmed" or "probable," and eliminated the date of onset criterion.[15] This standardized definition has subsequently been revised twice by the CSTE. In 2017, the description of acute onset weakness within the clinical criteria was changed from "focal" to "flaccid," and guidance regarding MRI results obtained within the first 72 hours after onset of weakness was provided.[17]

The most recent update released by the CSTE in June 2019 added additional MRI criteria to include any spinal cord lesion on MRI at least partially in the gray matter, excluding malignancy, vascular disease, or anatomic abnormalities. For a case to be classified as confirmed, the stipulation for "absence of a clear alternative diagnosis" was also added. Probable classification was expanded to include cases whereby gray matter predominance cannot be distinguished and the requirement for cerebrospinal fluid (CSF) pleocytosis was removed. Finally, the classification of "suspect" was included to capture cases lacking sufficient evidence to be designated as probable or confirmed.[18]

VIROLOGY

AFP surveillance conducted as part of the World Health Organization's strategy for polio eradication has led to advanced knowledge of the human enteroviruses (EVs), which comprise the largest genus of the picornavirus family.[3,19] EVs include poliovi-ruses, as well as the NPEVs, the first of which (coxsackievirus A1) was isolated in 1947 from a child with AFP.[3] NPEV infections manifest most commonly as mild ill-nesses but are also implicated in more severe, life-threatening conditions, such as myocarditis, encephalitis, meningitis, and possibly type 1 diabetes.[3,19] Some species of NPEVs have been observed to circulate in cyclic intervals. One such example is hu-man enterovirus 71 (EV-A71), which causes upticks of infections every 2 to 3 years in Southeast Asia.[3] Since 1988, multiple NPEVs have been linked to thousands of cases of AFP.[3] Surveillance analysis in the Philippines revealed that NPEVs accounted for about three-fourths of the total laboratory isolates from AFP patients between 1992 and 2008.[19]

EPIDEMIOLOGY AND VIRAL ASSOCIATION

Although AFP has been reported sporadically across the globe for decades, the dis-ease has only recently emerged in epidemic form in temporal association with EV-D68 outbreaks.[3] Van Haren and colleagues[20] examined the California epidemic with the reporting interval of June 2012 to July 2015, describing 59 cases meeting criteria for AFM out of more than 220 cases of neurologic illness investigated by the CDPH during this time period. Specimens yielding sequencing consistent with EV-D68 were obtained in 9 of these patients.[20]

The 11 AFM patients identified during the Colorado outbreak in 2014 were slightly younger (median age, 8 years), 73% were male cases, 91% had antecedent respira-tory symptoms, and EV-D68–positive specimens were obtained from 36%.[2] A retro-spective case-control study conducted by Aliabadi and colleagues[2] compared EV-D68 detected in the Colorado cluster AFM cases with 2 groups of controls who had mild respiratory illness. The findings demonstrated significantly higher incidence of EV-D68 identification in children with AFM over both groups of controls, supporting an epidemiologic association between EV-D68 and AFM.[2]

Among global reports of note, 59 cases of AFM were identified in Japan coincident with an EV-D68 national outbreak in autumn 2015.[21] Knoester and colleagues[22] re-ported EV-D68-associated AFM in patients from 12 different European countries iden-tified by a working group network in 2016. The investigators postulated that these 29 patients represented an underestimation of the total true cases of EV-D68–associated AFM in Europe because of late or absent testing.[22] In reports from Japan and Europe, most patients were children (median age, 4.4 and 4 years, respectively).[21,22] In cases whereby pathogens were isolated, respiratory samples were the most common means of pathogen detection.[21,22]

Nationwide surveillance using a standard case definition was instituted by the CDC in 2014. Since that time, 2 spikes of increasing magnitude have been recorded in the United States in the late summer/early fall of 2016 and 2018 as depicted in **Fig. 1**.[23,24] In the United States, 149 cases were confirmed by the CDC in 2016.[24] 2018 recorded the most cases to date with 233 confirmed cases across 41 states.[24] The median age reported for confirmed cases was 5.3 years (range, 6 months to 81.8 years), and 58% were male cases.[24]

Of the 233 confirmed cases of AFM in the United States in 2018, the CDC evaluated respiratory specimens in 123, yielding EV or rhinovirus in 44%. EV-A71 was the sec-ond most common pathogen isolated behind EV-D68 **(Fig. 2)**.[24] Messacar and

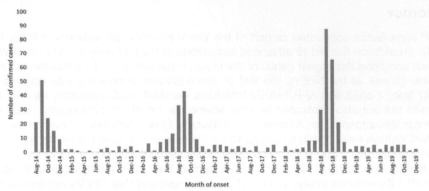

Fig. 1. Confirmed AFM cases by CDC from August 2014 through February 28, 2020, with onset of condition by December 31, 2019. (*From* Centers for Disease Control and Prevention, (CDC). AFM cases and outbreaks. https://www.cdc.gov/acute-flaccid-myelitis/cases-in-us. html.)

colleagues[25] examined a 2018 outbreak of EV-A71–associated neurologic disease characterized by fever, myoclonus, weakness, ataxia, and autonomic instability in children presenting to Children's Hospital Colorado. Their results indicated that children with EV-A71–associated AFM were more likely to present with a history of cutaneous lesions, displayed more ataxia, myoclonus, and irritability before weakness onset, had more generalized symmetric weakness, and were more likely to fully recover than children with EV-D68–associated AFM.[25]

The pathogenic process by which enteroviral infection results in AFM is not fully understood. Pathogens have proven difficult to isolate, and sites of injury (motor neurons in the spinal cord and bulbar gray) are not available for safe biopsy.[3] Changes in population immunity, viral evolution, and host susceptibility factors have been posited to explain the rare development of AFM in populations demonstrating widespread neutralizing antibodies to EV-D68.[3,26] Most studies have identified a male predominance in AFM.[20,27,28]

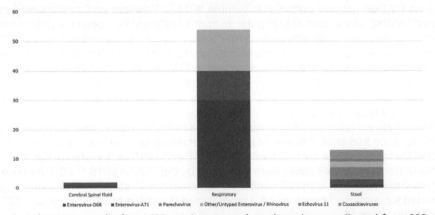

Fig. 2. Laboratory results from CSF, respiratory, and stool specimens collected from 233 patients with confirmed acute flaccid myelitis—United States, 2018. (*Data from* Lopez A, Lee A, Guo A, et al. Vital signs: surveillance for acute flaccid myelitis - United States, 2018. MMWR Morb Mortal Wkly Rep 2019;68:608-614.)

CLINICAL PRESENTATION

The typical presentation of AFM can be conceptualized in 3 stages: prodromal illness, acute, and convalescent (**Table 1**).[6,29,30] Most prodromal illnesses are characterized by fever (78% of confirmed cases in 2018) and respiratory tract symptoms (83%), such as cough, congestion, or rhinorrhea, although gastrointestinal symptoms, such as vomiting and diarrhea, may occur (36%).[24] As in cases of EV-A71–associated AFM, patients may present with hand, foot, and mouth lesions. The acute phase of AFM is heralded by the onset of focal weakness with hypotonia and hyporeflexia. In both the 2016 and the 2018 outbreaks, the median interval between prodrome and onset of weakness was 5 days, although this interval may extend up to 4 weeks.[24,29]

The pattern of weakness is typically monoplegia with asymmetric progression to multiple limbs, reaching nadir as rapidly as less than 6 hours or over the course of days.[6,10] Upper limbs tend to be more affected than lower limbs, proximal muscles more so than distal, with severity of weakness ranging from trace to complete paralysis.[4,10,29] Head and trunk control may be compromised in cases of generalized weakness.

Respiratory suppression is of ultimate concern and may progress rapidly. The CDC reported 27% of confirmed cases in 2018 required some type of respiratory support; of those, 87% required mechanical ventilation.[24] Cranial nerves, particularly VI, VII, IX, and X, may be affected leading to facial palsy, oromotor dysfunction, and pharyngeal dysphagia.[6,7,10]

Although AFM is thought to result from a pathogenic process that spares the sensory tracts, reports of pain in the affected extremities are common and have been reported to confound diagnosis.[4,7] Bowel and bladder dysfunction, including constipation, urinary retention, and incontinence, has been reported variably in cohorts, although incontinence may be difficult to precisely evaluate in young children.[4,10,29,30] Sensation is typically intact but has been reported to be abnormal in up to 25% of patients with AFM.[29] Once examination has stabilized and no new symptoms are being reported, patients may be considered to have entered the convalescent stage.[6] Over the course of months to years, patients in the convalescent stage may experience persistent weakness, atrophy, and acquired musculoskeletal deformities.[10,29]

Table 1		
Stages of clinical presentation in acute flaccid myelitis		
Prodrome	**Acute Neurologic Injury**	**Convalescent Stage**
• Fever (temperature ≥38°C) in nearly all patients	• Asymmetric onset of flaccid weakness in one or more limbs	• Variable recovery of motor function occurring distal → proximal
• Respiratory symptoms most common	○ Nadir after hours to days	• Complete recovery in minority of cases
○ Cough, sneezing, rhinorrhea	○ Monoplegia may progress to quadriplegia	• Musculoskeletal complications
• Possible symptoms	• Cranial nerve involvement possible	○ Hip subluxation or dislocation
○ Vomiting	○ Facial weakness	○ Contractures
○ Diarrhea	○ Dysphagia	○ Shoulder subluxation
○ Hand, foot, and mouth lesions	• Respiratory compromise common	○ Scoliosis
		○ Decreased bone mineral density and fractures
		○ Leg length discrepancy in developing children

IMAGING FINDINGS

MRI of the neuraxis is essential for diagnosis and should be obtained as soon as AFM is suspected. Longitudinal T2-weighted hyperintensity involving the central gray matter with edema is the characteristic feature.[30–32] In the acute stage, gray matter hyperintensities are frequently ill defined, bilateral, and extensive (>3 vertebral segments), with lack of gadolinium enhancement.[6,31] Over time, MRI lesions may become more sharply defined and display decreased longitudinal extension with greater selectivity for the anterior horns.[6,31,32] Extension into the white matter is not uncommonly reported, although extensive white matter involvement should prompt consideration of an alternative diagnosis, such as acute transverse myelitis, in the appropriate clinical setting.[9,30] White matter lesions noted acutely have been reported not to persist into the convalescent stage.[6] Nerve root enhancement, reported in the ventral cervical nerves and cauda equina, is most prominent after 1 to 2 weeks (**Fig. 3**).[31,32] Cranial MRI may show lesions in the cortical gray matter, dorsal pons, medulla oblongata, midbrain, and occasionally, the cerebellum.[6,7,31,32] Supratentorial white matter lesions are commonly noted in pediatric multiple sclerosis and acute disseminated encephalomyelitis; however, they are not a feature of AFM.[7,9]

LABORATORY TESTING

For any patient suspected of having AFM based on clinical and imaging criteria, the CDC requests that clinicians contact their local health department to provide clinical history and biologic specimens.[33] CSF, respiratory (nasopharyngeal [NP] or oropharyngeal [OP]) swabs, serum, and whole stool samples should be collected as close as possible to the onset of limb weakness and stored in accordance with the protocols outlined in the CDC's Job Aid for Clinicians (https://www.cdc.gov/acute-flaccid-myelitis/hcp/specimen-collection.html).[33] The CDC encourages prompt action, as data suggest earlier specimen collection has been associated with higher pathogen yield.[24]

Lumbar puncture for CSF analysis should be performed to exclude alternative diagnoses and to support the diagnosis of AFM. Typical CSF findings in AFM include lymphocytic pleocytosis with normal or elevated protein.[5,7,9] CSF pleocytosis is typically moderate (median white cell counts <100 per μL), although cell counts may be normal.[5,30] CSF culture and polymerase chain reaction (PCR) assays for EV RNA, herpes simplex virus, and varicella-zoster virus should be obtained, although they are negative in most AFM cases.[4,5,24] Mishra and colleagues[34] detected antibodies to human EVs using peptide microarray in the CSF of 79% of a cohort of 14 patients with AFM compared with 20% of controls with non-AFM CNS disease. This finding provides further indirect support for the role of EV infection in the pathogenesis of AFM and suggests an avenue for future investigation in diagnosis.[34]

Respiratory samples comprise the most frequent means by which pathogens are identified in AFM (see **Fig. 2**). NP and OP swabs for EV PCR as well as additional respiratory viruses (ie, rhinovirus and influenza) should be acquired in patients under suspicion for AFM.[4] Given that EV-D68 may only be detectable for the first 5 to 7 days of infection, negative respiratory results are common and should not preclude the diagnosis.[9,24,30]

Unlike polio, EV-D68 is not shed in stool. Stool samples should still be obtained in suspected AFM, as they may detect EV-A71, among other nonpolio viral pathogens.[4,9] In addition, stool samples continue to be assessed by the CDC for poliovirus in the United States given the potential for infection introduced by travelers or vaccine-derived neurovirulent strains.[4,35]

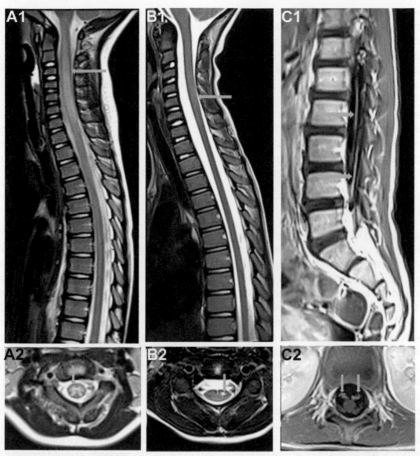

Fig. 3. (*A1*) Sagittal MRI obtained in a patient with acute AFM showing marked cervical cord edema. (*A2*) Axial image at C3 shows the T2 hyperintensity and edema centered on the gray matter. There was no enhancement during the acute stage in this patient. (*B1-2*) MRI obtained 3 months after recovery from AFM, T2 signal in most of the spinal cord normalized in this patient; however, asymmetric T2 hyperintensity of the anterior horns of the cervical cord persisted. (*C1-2*) A patient 2 months after onset of AFM. There is marked enhancement of the ventral nerve roots of the cauda equina. Acute images: Marked cervical cord edema. Axial image at C3 shows the T2 hyperintensity and edema is centered on the gray matter. There was no enhancement during the acute stage in this patient.

Additional serologies of utility to narrow the differential of AFP include antibodies against aquaporin-4 (AQP4), myelin oligodendrocyte protein (MOG), Lyme disease, and Epstein-Barr virus. The presence of AQP4 or MOG antibodies points toward demyelinating syndromes distinct from AFM.[9] Because West Nile virus has been reported in association with AFM, antibody assays for this pathogen in CSF and in serum should be considered when seasonally and geographically appropriate.[4]

ELECTRODIAGNOSTIC FINDINGS

Electromyography (EMG) and nerve conduction studies (NCS) are not obligatory investigations for AFM but may provide valuable diagnostic clarity in certain cases. NCS typically show decreased amplitude or absence of compound muscle action potentials (CMAPs), diminished or absent F-waves, normal motor conduction velocity, normal distal motor latencies, and preserved sensory nerve action potentials (SNAPs) **(Table 2)**.[30,36–38] Needle EMG examination of affected muscles may reveal absent or reduced recruitment of motor unit action potentials (MUAPs) with evidence of sub-acute denervation (positive sharp waves and fibrillations) and/or chronic neurogenic changes (enlarged, polyphasic MUAPs).[5,36–38] As has been well documented in polio-myelitis, spontaneous activity (positive sharp waves and fibrillations) in AFM may be more prominent 4 to 6 weeks after the onset of weakness.[38] This overall electrodiag-nostic picture of an isolated motor neuropathic process with axon loss and sparing of sensory nerves may be of particular utility in distinguishing AFM from an inflammatory peripheral neuropathy.[7] Electrodiagnostic testing also has utility for preoperative plan-ning of nerve or tendon transfer for the treatment of AFM.[39]

ACUTE TREATMENT

Hospitalization is indicated for any patient presenting with signs and symptoms concern-ing for AFM with close monitoring for respiratory compromise and autonomic insta-bility.[7,24] Intensive care admission may be necessitated, particularly for those with increased risk for deterioration on the basis of upper-extremity weakness and bulbar symptoms.[4] Neurology and infectious disease specialists should be consulted promptly. The CDC Web site features a link to assist clinicians managing suspected cases of AFM with consulting specialists affiliated with the University of Texas Southwestern's Trans-verse Myelitis Center or Johns Hopkins University Transverse Myelitis Center (https://myelitis.org/living-with-myelitis/resources/afm-physician-support-portal).[8]

No prospective, controlled clinical trials have been completed to date upon which to base recommendations for specific therapies in AFM.[8,9] Treatments in common use include single administration or combinations of intravenous immunoglobulin (IVIg), intravenous corticosteroids, plasma exchange (PLEX), fluoxetine, and antiviral agents. Rationale for IVIg in AFM is supported by laboratory data, confirming high levels of neutralizing antibodies against EV-D68 in commercially available lots as well as its uti-lization in the treatment of enteroviral infection in pediatric patients with agammaglob-ulinemia.[9,40] Although expensive, IVIg is generally safe and well tolerated. Prevaccine trials against poliomyelitis as well as recent studies in a mouse model of EV-D68–asso-ciated AFM suggest efficacy of IVIg; however, therapeutic benefit appears to diminish with administration later in the disease course.[8,9,41] Given that patients with AFM typi-cally develop weakness days to weeks after infection, the time sensitivity of IVIg treat-ment initiation may account for the lack of clear disease modification reflected in the limited available literature.[8,9]

The edema and white matter inflammation observed in AFM lend theoretic justifica-tion for corticosteroid treatment, which is considered to be first line for other causes of inflammatory myelitis.[8,9] Objections to steroid therapy in AFM center on the implica-tions of immunosuppression in a process that is favored to be the result, at least in part, of direct viral neuronal cytotoxicity. Aside from the absence of clinical data sup-porting efficacy, there is evidence that steroids exacerbate neuroinvasive disease in NPEVs; and steroids were demonstrated to increase mortality and worsen paralysis in the mouse model of AFM.[7,8,41]

PLEX has also been used in combination with other therapies in the treatment of AFM. No studies have evaluated PLEX monotherapy. In addition to the requirement for invasive vascular access and insufficient evidence of benefit, concerns have been raised that PLEX may potentiate the disease process by removing antibodies involved in the immune response to enteroviral infection.[8]

Table 2
Summary of electrodiagnostic findings in acute flaccid myelitis

	NCS					EMG	
CMAP	Motor Conduction Velocity	Distal Motor Latency	SNAP	F-wave		MUAP	Spontaneous Activity
Decreased amplitude or absent	Normal (if obtainable)	Normal (if obtainable)	Normal	Diminished or absent		• May be volitionally absent • Reduced recruitment • Enlarged/polyphasic	• Positive sharp waves/fibrillation • May be present acutely and more prominent over time

Fluoxetine has been proposed as a treatment for AFM based on demonstrated inhibition of EV-D68 replication in vitro.[42] Messacar and colleagues[43] retrospectively evaluated a multicenter cohort of 56 AFM patients, 30 of whom had been administered fluoxetine a median of 5 days after the onset of neurologic symptoms. This study concluded that although well tolerated, fluoxetine did not improve neurologic outcomes compared with untreated patients.[43] Fluoxetine also failed to improve motor outcomes or reduce viral titers in the mouse model of EV-D68–associated AFM.[41]

The antiviral agents, pleconaril, pocapavir, and vapendavir, have been assessed by the CDC for in vitro activity against EV-D68 with negative results, although protease inhibitors have shown promise in laboratory experiments.[8,44] Currently, the CDC does not endorse the use of antiviral agents in AFM, exempting cases in which herpesvirus infection is suspected.[8] Appropriate antivirals should be empirically continued in the acute setting until herpesvirus infection has been ruled out.[8]

NERVE TRANSFER SURGERIES

Nerve transfer surgeries aim to restore voluntary movement by using working nerves as a motor source for denervated muscles. To mitigate donor deficit, nerves serving muscles where there is redundancy in a particular joint function (ie, elbow flexion) are typically selected.[39] In peripheral nerve lesions, such as brachial plexopathy, this technique is an accepted treatment and has been proposed in AFM patients with persistent flaccid paralysis after 6 to 9 months.[11,39]

Pino and colleagues[11] conducted a retrospective case analysis of 11 patients with AFM who had undergone nerve transfers with at least 6 months of documented follow-up. Common recipients included the musculocutaneous, radial branch to triceps, suprascapular, and axillary nerves. Excellent recovery, which was defined as full antigravity motion, was noted in 87% of patients for elbow flexion and 67% for elbow extension. Recovery of shoulder function was less promising, with excellent recovery of external rotation in 50% and abduction in only 20%. Notably, 90% of patients with transfers to the suprascapular nerve had resolution of shoulder subluxation.[11]

Owing to the progressive motor endplate degeneration that occurs in chronically denervated muscles, a presently undefined window of opportunity may exist for nerve transfer surgery in AFM. Doi and colleagues[45] reported 1 case of successful restoration of quadricep function after contralateral obturator nerve transfer in a 7-year-old boy with AFM. This same procedure achieved unsatisfactory quadricep strength in 3 subsequent patients, which the investigators note underwent surgery greater than 12 months after the onset of weakness, suggesting that early referral may be preferential.[45] Although the study by Pino and colleagues[11] included 2 patients who underwent surgery after 15 months from onset of AFM and had comparable results to the remainder of the cohort, the investigators recommend early surgical referral given that delayed nerve transfer has been associated with worse outcomes in neonatal brachial plexus palsies.[46]

REHABILITATION

Early initiation of intensive rehabilitation with multidisciplinary therapy services to include physical therapy (PT), occupational therapy (OT), and speech therapy has been advocated for the treatment of AFM.[3,4,9,47] Melicosta and colleagues[10] described the rehabilitation and medical management of a cohort of 31 patients (14 outpatient and 17 inpatient) with AFM participating in an intensive activity based restorative therapy (ABRT) program at a single pediatric center. The patients admitted to acute rehabilitation for ABRT received PT, OT, and speech therapy services with additional consultations (ie, respiratory therapy, nutrition) used in accordance with the individual needs of the child (age range, 7 months to 16 years old).[10] Notable components of ABRT include functional electrical stimulation, weight-supported locomotion and weight bearing, and task-specific practice.[10] Rehabilitative outcomes measured by standardized assessments (Spinal Cord Injury Measure, Physical Ability and Mobility Scale, and the Functional Independence Measure for Children) suggested ABRT resulted in functional benefit, even when initiated years after diagnosis.[10]

Of patients who necessitated ventilatory support on admission, 80% were discharged with decreased requirements (lower mechanical ventilator settings, positive airway pressure only during the day, or liberation from the ventilator).[10] Ability to wean ventilation was associated with older age and shorter interval between onset of AFM and admission to rehabilitation.[10] Two patients in this cohort had undergone diaphragmatic pacing, which was associated with only slight benefits.[10] A single case report describing implantation of a direct diaphragmatic pacing system in a 3-year-old girl with AFM 3 weeks after presentation reported improved respiratory function reflected by decreased ventilator support and improved hemidiaphragmatic excursion.[48] Although this patient did not achieve complete liberation from the ventilator, early implantation of pacers before advanced atrophy and fibrosis of the diaphragm occurs is postulated to enhance success.[10,48] Thoracoscopic intercostal nerve to phrenic nerve transfer has also been performed in patients with AFM.[11]

Bowel and bladder function should be assessed in rehabilitation with regimens for management instituted as appropriate. Urinary and/or bowel incontinence and constipation have been variably reported and may be more prominent acutely.[10,27,47] Recalling that sensorium is typically unaltered in AFM, bowel and bladder dysfunction may not only cause pain and discomfort but also potentiate dysautonomia.[47]

Patients confronted with sudden disability, often profound, resulting from AFM may experience anxiety, depression, and adjustment disorder.[47,49] Social workers, behavioral psychologists, child life specialists, and recreational therapists are valuable members of the rehabilitation team in providing psychosocial assessments and support and should be readily consulted. The Acute Flaccid Myelitis Association provides advocacy and support for affected patients and families, including a list of rehabilitation facilities with experience in treating patients with AFM (www.afmanow.org).[50]

OUTCOMES

Although the literature pertaining to recovery in AFM is variable, prognosis is generally regarded to be poor with most children suffering persistent functional deficits. Return of motor function typically begins distally, and despite therapy, many patients are bothered by chronic weakness and wasting of the proximal limb muscles.[6,10,13] Full clinical recovery was reported in only 10% of patients in the cohort of EV-D68–associated AFM described by Knoester and colleagues,[22] which also included 2 fatalities. Kane and colleagues[28] reported full recovery in 41% of 28 AFM patients from Northern California. More promising reports of complete recovery may be attributable to the inclusion of less severe cases as well as non-D68 enteroviral infections, such as the prognostically favorable EV-A71.[25,28] Recovery appears to be most robust within the first 12 months after onset; however, continued progress has been seen up to 18 months of follow-up.[13]

Some studies have explored the association between advanced imaging findings and clinical manifestations in AFM. Okumura and colleagues[31] reviewed MRI results in 54 children with AFM associated with the 2015 EV-D68 outbreak in Japan, finding no relationship between outcome and the extent, localization, or appearance of spinal lesions on advanced imaging. McCoy and colleagues[51] examined cervical MRI findings in 9 AFM patients and reported a correlation between clinical disability and percentage of gray matter axial T2 signal hyperintensity at the most affected spinal level. Martin and colleagues[12] reported incongruency between clinical outcome and follow-up MRI obtained months after diagnosis, in contrast to EMG/NCS findings, which displayed a correlation between the degree of electrodiagnostic abnormalities and ongoing weakness.

SUMMARY

AFM is an incompletely understood syndrome of flaccid paralysis, predominately affecting children, preceded by acute infectious symptoms and identified by lesions involving the spinal cord gray matter. Although several treatments have been used in an attempt to halt or limit neurologic damage occurring during the acute phase of the disease, none have presently been proven effective, leaving most affected individuals with lasting impairments. There is substantial heterogeneity in the clinical presentation, pattern, and severity of paralysis, and trajectory of recovery for various patients, necessitating a tailored, individualized approach to rehabilitation. Employment of a skilled multidisciplinary rehabilitation team to address AFM's extensive and often profound impacts on a patient's mobility, respiratory status, autonomic function, communication, social interaction, and mental health is essential.

Significant gaps in the current knowledge of AFM persist in every aspect of the disease. Literature interpretation is confounded by a broad and evolving epidemiologic case definition, which has been engineered to optimize reporting rather than provide clinical diagnostic precision. An understanding of known epidemiology, characteristics, workup, therapies, and potential alternative diagnoses is nevertheless necessary to best equip providers combating AFM and its long-term sequelae. Pediatric and adult rehabilitation physicians are uniquely positioned to observe the course of AFM, scrutinize interventions, and strive to maximize function for years to come.

CLINICS CARE POINTS

- Acute flaccid myelitis causes motor impairment affecting limbs, cranial nerves, and respiratory musculature with variation in severity and pattern of involvement.

- Advanced imaging in the acute phase will typically show longitudinally extensive gray matter lesions that become more localized to the anterior horns in the convalescent stage. White matter involvement, if present acutely, typically resolves with time.

- Electrodiagnostic results will be consistent with motor neuropathy/neuronopathy with normal sensory nerve conduction studies, although up to 25% of patients report impaired sensation.

- Management is supportive. More research is needed to establish effective disease-modifying therapy in the acute setting.

- Early initiation of comprehensive therapies is recommended to restore function and mitigate chronic complications; however, functional gains can still be achieved months to years after onset.

- Referral for nerve transfer surgery may be considered for patients with persistent paralysis. Early research suggests surgery may be most effective in restoring elbow flexion and reducing shoulder subluxation.

- Determination of long-term outcomes for acute flaccid myelitis will require continued research.

- Most patients will have persistent functional deficits and benefit from ongoing rehabilitation services for therapies, mobility equipment, bracing, orthopedic surveillance, and psychosocial support.

DISCLOSURE

The authors have nothing to disclose.

REFERENCES

1. Ayscue P, Van Haren K, Sheriff H, et al. Acute flaccid paralysis with anterior myelitis—California, June 2012–June 2014. MMWR Morb Mortal Wkly Rep 2014;63(40):903.
2. Aliabadi N, Messacar K, Pastula DM, et al. Enterovirus D68 infection in children with acute flaccid myelitis, Colorado, USA, 2014. Emerg Infect Dis 2016;22(8): 1387.
3. Morens DM, Folkers GK, Fauci AS. Acute flaccid myelitis: something old and something new. MBio 2019;10(2):521.
4. Hopkins SE, Elrick MJ, Messacar K. Acute flaccid myelitis—keys to diagnosis, questions about treatment, and future directions. JAMA Pediatr 2019;173(2): 117–8.
5. Elrick MJ, Gordon-Lipkin E, Crawford TO, et al. Clinical subpopulations in a sample of North American children diagnosed with acute flaccid myelitis, 2012-2016. JAMA Pediatr 2019;173(2):134–9.
6. Gordon-Lipkin E, Muñoz LS, Klein JL, et al. Comparative quantitative clinical, neuroimaging, and functional profiles in children with acute flaccid myelitis at acute and convalescent stages of disease. Dev Med Child Neurol 2019;61(3):366–75.
7. Hopkins SE. Acute flaccid myelitis: etiologic challenges, diagnostic and management considerations. Curr Treat Options Neurol 2017;19(12):48.
8. Centers for Disease Control and Prevention, (CDC). Acute flaccid myelitis: interim considerations for clinical management. Available at: https://www.cdc.gov/acute-flaccid-myelitis/hcp/clinical-management.html. Accessed March 25, 2020.
9. Theroux LM, Brenton JN. Acute transverse and flaccid myelitis in children. Curr Treat Options Neurol 2019;21(12):64.
10. Melicosta ME, Dean J, Hagen K, et al. Acute flaccid myelitis: rehabilitation challenges and outcomes in a pediatric cohort. J Pediatr Rehabil Med 2019;12(3): 245–53.
11. Pino PA, Intravia J, Kozin SH, et al. Early results of nerve transfers for restoring function in severe cases of acute flaccid myelitis. Ann Neurol 2019;86(4):607–15.
12. Martin JA, Messacar K, Yang ML, et al. Outcomes of Colorado children with acute flaccid myelitis at 1 year. Neurology 2017;89(2):129–37.
13. Kirolos A, Mark K, Shetty J, et al. Outcome of paediatric acute flaccid myelitis associated with enterovirus D68: a case series. Dev Med Child Neurol 2019; 61(3):376–80.
14. Centers for Disease Control and Prevention, (CDC). For clinicians: diagnosing acute flaccid myelitis (AFM) in the United States. Available at: https://www.cdc.gov/acute-flaccid-myelitis/downloads/afm-presentation.pdf. Accessed March 29, 2020.
15. Council of State and Territorial Epidemiologists, (CSTE). Standardized case definition for acute flaccid myelitis. Available at: https://cdn.ymaws.com/www.cste.

org/resource/resmgr/2015PS/2015PSFinal/15-ID-01.pdf. Accessed March 25, 2020.

16. Centers for Disease Control and Prevention, (CDC). Acute flaccid myelitis (AFM) 2020 case definition. Available at: https://wwwn.cdc.gov/nndss/conditions/acute-flaccid-myelitis/case-definition/2020/. Accessed March 23, 2020.

17. Council of State and Territorial Epidemiologists, (CSTE). Revision to the standardized surveillance and case definition for acute flaccid myelitis. Available at: https://cdn.ymaws.com/www.cste.org/resource/resmgr/2017PS/2017PSFinal/17-ID-01.pdf. Accessed March 25, 2020.

18. Council of State and Territorial Epidemiologists, (CSTE). Revision to the standardized case definition, case classification, and public health reporting for acute flaccid myelitis. Available at: https://cdn.ymaws.com/www.cste.org/resource/resmgr/2019ps/final/19-ID-05_AFM_final_7.31.19.pdf. Accessed March 25, 2020.

19. Apostol LN, Suzuki A, Bautista A, et al. Detection of non-polio enteroviruses from 17 years of virological surveillance of acute flaccid paralysis in the Philippines. J Med Virol 2012;84(4):624–31.

20. Van Haren K, Ayscue P, Waubant E, et al. Acute flaccid myelitis of unknown etiology in California, 2012-2015. JAMA 2015;314(24):2663–71.

21. Chong PF, Kira R, Mori H, et al. Clinical features of acute flaccid myelitis temporally associated with an enterovirus D68 outbreak: results of a nationwide survey of acute flaccid paralysis in Japan, August-December 2015. Clin Infect Dis 2018; 66(5):653–64.

22. Knoester M, Helfferich J, Poelman R, et al. Twenty-nine cases of enterovirus-D68-associated acute flaccid myelitis in Europe 2016: a case series and epidemiologic overview. Pediatr Infect Dis J 2019;38(1):16.

23. Centers for Disease Control and Prevention, (CDC). AFM cases and outbreaks. Available at: https://www.cdc.gov/acute-flaccid-myelitis/cases-in-us.html. Accessed March 27, 2020.

24. Lopez A. Vital signs: surveillance for acute flaccid myelitis - United States, 2018. MMWR Morb Mortal Wkly Rep 2019;68:608–14.

25. Messacar K, Spence-Davizon E, Osborne C, et al. Clinical characteristics of enterovirus A71 neurological disease during an outbreak in children in Colorado, USA, in 2018: an observational cohort study. Lancet Infect Dis 2020;20(2):230–9.

26. Kamau E, Harvala H, Blomqvist S, et al. Increase in enterovirus D68 infections in young children, United Kingdom, 2006–2016. Emerg Infect Dis 2019;25(6):1200.

27. Messacar K, Schreiner TL, Van Haren K, et al. Acute flaccid myelitis: a clinical review of US cases 2012–2015. Ann Neurol 2016;80(3):326–38.

28. Kane MS, Sonne C, Zhu S, et al. Incidence, risk factors and outcomes among children with acute flaccid myelitis: a population-based cohort study in a California health network between 2011 and 2016. Pediatr Infect Dis J 2019;38(7): 667–72.

29. Fatemi Y, Chakraborty R. Acute flaccid myelitis: a clinical overview for 2019. Mayo Clin Proc 2019;94(5):875–81.

30. Murphy OC, Pardo CA. Acute flaccid myelitis: a clinical review. Semin Neurol 2020;40(2):211–8.

31. Okumura A, Mori H, Chong PF, et al. Serial MRI findings of acute flaccid myelitis during an outbreak of enterovirus D68 infection in Japan. Brain Dev 2019;41(5): 443–51.

32. Maloney JA, Mirsky DM, Messacar K, et al. MRI findings in children with acute flaccid paralysis and cranial nerve dysfunction occurring during the 2014 enterovirus D68 outbreak. AJNR Am J Neuroradiol 2015;36(2):245–50.
33. Centers for Disease Control and Prevention, (CDC). Acute flaccid myelitis (AFM): data collection. 2020. Available at: https://www.cdc.gov/acute-flaccid-myelitis/hcp/data-collection.html. Accessed April 5, 2020.
34. Mishra N, Ng TFF, Marine RL, et al. Antibodies to enteroviruses in cerebrospinal fluid of patients with acute flaccid myelitis. MBio 2019;10(4):1903.
35. Jorba J, Diop OM, Iber J, et al. Update on vaccine-derived poliovirus outbreak - worldwide, January-June 2019. MMWR Morb Mortal Wkly Rep 2019;68(45):1024.
36. Andersen EW, Kornberg AJ, Freeman JL, et al. Acute flaccid myelitis in childhood: a retrospective cohort study. Eur J Neurol 2017;24(8):1077–83.
37. Patel R, Goyal P, Verma S. Clinical, radiological and electrodiagnostic (EMG/NCS) profile in acute flaccid myelitis (AFM). Neurology 2017;88(16 Supplement):P6.115.
38. Hovden IAH, Pfeiffer HCV. Electrodiagnostic findings in acute flaccid myelitis related to enterovirus D68. Muscle Nerve 2015;52(5):909–10.
39. Saltzman EB, Rancy SK, Sneag DB, et al. Nerve transfers for enterovirus D68-associated acute flaccid myelitis: a case series. Pediatr Neurol 2018;88:25–30. Available at: http://www.sciencedirect.com/science/article/pii/S0887899417311360.
40. Zhang Y, Moore DD, Nix WA, et al. Neutralization of enterovirus D68 isolated from the 2014 US outbreak by commercial intravenous immune globulin products. J Clin Virol 2015;69:172–5.
41. Hixon AM, Clarke P, Tyler KL. Evaluating treatment efficacy in a mouse model of enterovirus D68–associated paralytic myelitis. J Infect Dis 2017;216(10):1245–53.
42. Tyler KL. Rationale for the evaluation of fluoxetine in the treatment of enterovirus D68-associated acute flaccid myelitis. JAMA Neurol 2015;72(5):493–4.
43. Messacar K, Sillau S, Hopkins SE, et al. Safety, tolerability, and efficacy of fluoxetine as an antiviral for acute flaccid myelitis. Neurology 2019;92(18):e2118–26.
44. Rhoden E, Zhang M, Nix WA, et al. In vitro efficacy of antiviral compounds against enterovirus D68. Antimicrob Agents Chemother 2015;59(12):7779–81.
45. Doi K, Sem SH, Hattori Y, et al. Contralateral obturator nerve to femoral nerve transfer for restoration of knee extension after acute flaccid myelitis: a case report. JBJS Case Connect 2019;9(4):e0073.
46. Little KJ, Zlotolow DA, Soldado F, et al. Early functional recovery of elbow flexion and supination following median and/or ulnar nerve fascicle transfer in upper neonatal brachial plexus palsy. J Bone Joint Surg Am 2014;96(3):215–21.
47. Hardy D, Hopkins S. Update on acute flaccid myelitis: recognition, reporting, aetiology and outcomes. Arch Dis Child 2020;105(9):842–7.
48. Edmiston TL, Elrick MJ, Kovler ML, et al. Early use of an implantable diaphragm pacing stimulator for a child with severe acute flaccid myelitis—a case report. Spinal Cord Ser Cases 2019;5(1):1–6.
49. Kornafel T, Tsao EY, Sabelhaus E, et al. Physical and occupational therapy for a teenager with acute flaccid myelitis: a case report. Phys Occup Ther Pediatr 2017;37(5):485–595.
50. Acute flaccid myelitis association. Available at: https://www.afmanow.org. Accessed April 25, 2020.
51. McCoy DB, Talbott JF, Wilson M, et al. MRI atlas-based measurement of spinal cord injury predicts outcome in acute flaccid myelitis. AJNR Am J Neuroradiol 2017;38(2):410–7.

Approach to Fatigue and Energy Conservation

Check for updates

Beth Grill, PT, DPT*, Maria Cole, OTR, MHA

KEYWORDS

- Fatigue • Energy conservation • Pacing • Postpolio syndrome

KEY POINTS

- Fatigue is one of the most debilitating complaints of individuals with postpolio syndrome (PPS).
- Medical management is critical to identify treatable comorbidities that may cause fatigue with PPS.
- Intervention for fatigue includes education on energy conservation, pacing, compensatory strategies, and equipment with PPS.
- A multidisciplinary approach is needed to manage the multifactorial components of fatigue in individuals with PPS.

INTRODUCTION: HISTORY, DEFINITIONS, AND BACKGROUND

Postpolio syndrome (PPS) is a slow, progressive lower motor neuron condition characterized by generalized fatigue, muscular fatigue, new onset of muscle weakness and atrophy, muscle and joint pain, cold intolerance, and new breathing and swallowing difficulties. Symptoms often interfere with an individual's quality of life, including participation in daily activities, work, and recreation.[1,2] After a period of relative stability, 15% to 80% of all people with poliomyelitis develop PPS depending on the population studied and criteria used.[3,4] Because there is no specific test, the diagnosis of PPS is made by exclusion using clinical criteria. The March of Dimes (MoD) criteria is broadly accepted (**Box 1**).[3,5]

Individuals with PPS report fatigue as the most common and incapacitating symptom at an incidence of 34% to 87%.[6] *Taber's Medical Dictionary* defines fatigue as "an overwhelming sustained feeling of exhaustion and diminished capacity for physical and mental work."[7] In the context of health and disease, there are many ways to categorize fatigue subtypes. Classification by the source of fatigue is one approach.[8]

Peripheral fatigue is defined as physical limitation related to failure of the peripheral nervous system (neuromuscular junction, muscles, and nerves) to sustain a level of activity or force.[8] Central fatigue occurs in the central nervous system (CNS) causing a

Spaulding Outpatient Center Framingham, 570 Worcester Road, Framingham, MA 01702, USA
* Corresponding author.
E-mail address: bgrill@partners.org

Phys Med Rehabil Clin N Am 32 (2021) 493–507
https://doi.org/10.1016/j.pmr.2021.02.011
1047-9651/21/© 2021 Elsevier Inc. All rights reserved.

Box 1
March of Dimes criteria for postpolio syndrome

1. Prior paralytic poliomyelitis with evidence of motor neuron loss, as confirmed by a history of the acute paralytic illness, signs of residual weakness and atrophy of muscles on neurologic examination, and signs of denervation on electromyography

2. A period of partial or complete functional recovery acute paralytic poliomyelitis, followed by an interval (usually 15 years or more) of stable neurologic function

3. Gradual or sudden onset of progressive and persistent weakness or abnormal muscle fatigability (decreased endurance), with or without generalized fatigue, muscle atrophy, or muscle and joint pain. (Sudden onset may follow a period of inactivity, or trauma, or surgery.) Less commonly, symptoms attributed to PPS include new problems with swallowing or breathing

4. Symptoms persisting for at least a year

5. Exclusion of other neurologic, medical, and orthopedic problems as causes of symptoms

Data from March of Dimes International Conference on Post-Polio Syndrome Identifying Best Practices in Diagnosis & Care. Published online May 19, 2000. Accessed August 2, 2020. https://www.polioplace.org/sites/default/files/files/MOD-%20Identifying.pdf.

---

progressive decline in motor neuron impulse transmission.[8] Mental fatigue involves difficulty with planning, concentration, and mental sustainability. Individuals with PPS who report fatigue may experience difficulty with initiating or sustaining physical activity and/or attentional tasks.[8] Although it is unclear if generalized fatigue reported by an individual with PPS is physiologic or multifactorial, it is important to consider all possible causes.[9]

In a small study of individuals reporting high levels of fatigue, MRI findings suggest that the polio virus affects the reticular activating system and additional CNS structures,[10] consistent with a postmortem study performed 50 to 70 years earlier.[9–11] Additional studies found evidence of noninfectious inflammation present in the spinal cord and peripheral blood; antibody responses; and increased levels of inflammatory cytokines in the cerebrospinal fluid.[3,6,9] These findings may contribute to central fatigue. At the neuromuscular level, the consensus is that ongoing denervation and reinnervation of the enlarged motor unit (up to 10 times larger than normal) are unable to compensate; thus, loss of motor units ensues.[3] The loss of motor units may contribute to peripheral muscle weakness and pain. Studies identified a circadian variation of fatigue in individuals with paralytic polio and PPS.[12,13] Sleep disorders, periodic leg movement, and respiratory muscle weakness are common in this population and may contribute to fatigue.[14] In addition, a decline in participation and function may contribute to affective mental fatigue.[8] According to Tersteeg,[6] fatigue is associated with physical and psychosocial variables, which include physical function, pain, sleep disorders, and mental health and task-oriented coping.

It is important to identify all causes of fatigue in individuals with PPS in order to provide pharmacologic and nonpharmacologic intervention. In conjunction, an individualized multidisciplinary approach to treatment is essential. Because fatigue in individuals with PPS is multifactorial, it is critical to address all confounding factors to ensure comprehensive care and positive outcomes.

The *aim* of this article is to

1. Identify causes of fatigue in individuals with PPS
2. Identify self-reported and performance-based outcome measure tools to assess fatigue in individuals with PPS

3. Recognize the role of energy conservation and pacing techniques in the management of fatigue with PPS
4. Apply the concepts of fatigue management to a case

DISCUSSION
Medical Work-Up

The medical work-up is critical to rule out causes of fatigue that are not related to PPS and provide appropriate intervention. Identifying the key factors in individuals with PPS is essential to identifying the correct pharmacologic and nonpharmacologic interventions (**Fig. 1**).[11,15] For example, compensatory movement patterns during ambulation in the setting of muscle weakness and joint degeneration may contribute to reduced movement efficiency and pain, which contribute to fatigue. Pain and fatigue should not be viewed as a natural part of aging in individuals with PPS.[16]

Sleep-related complaints are present in nearly half of all individuals with PPS.[14] Clinical symptoms of sleep-disordered breathing include excessive daytime somnolence (progressive worsening of fatigue in the afternoon), insomnia, snoring, morning

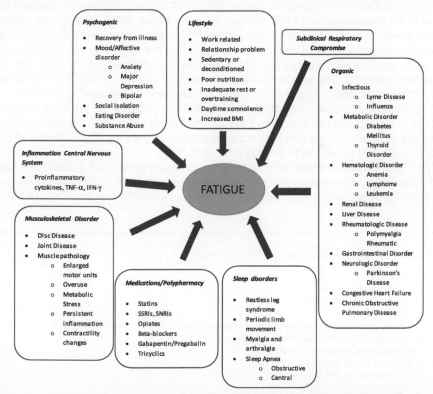

Fig. 1. Causes of fatigue adapted for PPS. The multifactorial causes impacting fatigue in individuals with PPS. BMI, body mass index; SNRIs, serotonin and norepinephrine reuptake inhibitors; SSRIs, selective serotonin reuptake inhibitors. (*Adapted from* Stacey Li Hi Shing, Rangariroyashe H. Chipika, Eoin Finegan, Deirdre Murray, Orla Hardiman, and Peter Bede. Post-polio Syndrome: More Than Just a Lower Motor Neuron Disease. Front. Neurol., 16 July 2019 https://doi.org/10.3389/fneur.2019.00773 and From The Rheumatology Book 2020 © Family Practice Notebook, LLC.)

headaches, cognitive manifestations, and fatigue.[14] Sleep-disordered breathing impedes ventilation through 3 different mechanisms: respiratory muscles weakness, upper airway resistance, and impaired central control. An additional factor may include skeletal trunk deformities, which contribute to decreased lung volume. Sleep-related movement disorders are seen frequently (63%) in individuals with polio sequelae. Restless leg syndrome (RLS) is a sensory motor disorder, whereas periodic leg movement, associated with RLS, may have a greater impact on cardiovascular risk.[14] Tersteeg[6] found a correlation with sleep quality and fatigue in individuals with PPS. The progressive and variable nature of PPS combined with bulbar involvement may explain the wide range of sleep-disorder breathing patterns seen with this population.[14] Given the prevalence and consequences of sleep disorders in individuals with PPS, systematic screening and referral to a sleep specialist with experience treating polio survivors are recommended. Furthermore, treatment of sleep disorders with nocturnal ventilation (CPAP, BiPAP) may improve fatigue.[14] The medical work-up may include the following laboratory testing to rule out other causes of fatigue[15] (**Box 2**).

Tests and Measures

Self-Reported Outcome Fatigue Scales aid in the measurement of fatigue.[17–19] Horemans and colleagues[20] examined reproducibility of 4 questionnaires to measure fatigue in 65 individuals with PPS: Fatigue Severity Scale (FSS), Nottingham Health Profile energy category, postpolio problem list (PPL) fatigue item, and Dutch Short Fatigue Questionnaire (SFQ). The findings revealed that the 4 questionnaires measured the same unidimensional construct with moderate reproducibility of the FSS, PPL fatigue item, and SFQ. The smallest detectable change was 1.5 for the FSS, 2.0 for the PPL fatigue item, and 1.9 for the SFQ. Vasconcelos and colleagues[17] compared the FFS, Fatigue Impact Scale, and Visual Analogue Scale (VAS) for fatigue in 56 subjects with 39 of those fitting the criteria for PPS. Of the 3 scales, the FSS was the strongest predictor of severe fatigue with moderate correlation to the VAS. The limitation of the FSS is it reduced sensitivity to change over time.[18]

The FSS is a self-administered questionnaire originally developed in 1989 by Krupp and colleagues[21] to measure disabling fatigue in patients with multiple sclerosis and systemic lupus erythematosus (**Box 3**). The FSS consists of 9 statements rated on a

---

Box 2
Medical work-up adapted for postpolio syndrome

Laboratory testing
A. Complete blood count
  a. Consider serum ferritin
  b. Consider B12
B. C-reactive protein or erythrocyte sedimentation rate
  a. Consider antinuclear antibody if abnormal
C. Comprehensive metabolic panel
  a. Includes serum glucose
  b. Includes serum electrolytes
  c. Includes renal function testing
  d. Includes liver function tests
D. Serum phosphorus
E. Thyroid-stimulating hormone
F. Urinalysis

Data from Moses S. Fatigue. Family Practice Notebook. Accessed August 9, 2020. https://fpnotebook.com/Rheum/Sx/FtgDgnstcTstng.htm.

Box 3
Fatigue Severity Scale (this is an outcome measure)

1. My motivation is lower when I am fatigued.
2. Exercise brings on my fatigue.
3. I am easily fatigued.
4. Fatigue interferes with my physical function.
5. Fatigue causes frequent problems for me.
6. My fatigue prevents sustained physical functioning.
7. Fatigue interferes with carrying out certain duties and responsibilities.
8. Fatigue is among my 3 most disabling symptoms.
9. Fatigue interferes with my work, family, or social life.

Data from Krupp LB, LaRocca NG, Muir-Nash J, Steinberg AD. The fatigue severity scale. Application to patients with multiple sclerosis and systemic lupus erythematosus. Arch Neurol. 1989;46(10):1121-1123.

7-point scale (1 = strongly disagree and 7 = strongly agree). A score is calculated as the mean of the 9 items, and ≥4 indicates a moderate to high level of fatigue.[18,22]

The FSS measures fatigue and non-fatigue-related concepts in "body functions" and "activities and participation" (**Fig. 2**). It is important to measure levels of fatigue and how fatigue impacts individuals with PPS in their daily life in order to identify appropriate interventions. The FSS, however, lacks sensitivity to detect real change beyond measurement error in a single subject following an intervention. It was found to be reliable and without floor or ceiling effect.[18]

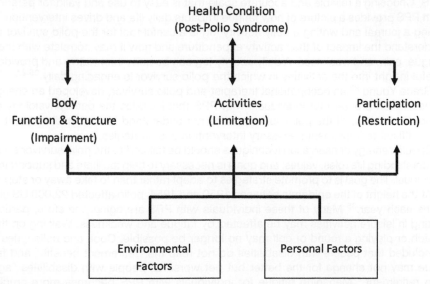

Fig. 2. The WHO-ICF model provides a framework for a common language in research and knowledge translation. (*From* International Classifications of Functioning, Disability and Health (ICF). World Health Organization. Published May 2001. Accessed August 16, 2020. https://www.who.int/classifications/icf/en/.)

Intervention

Energy conservation and pacing

When I consult my doctors, they bring me their knowledge of medicine to the conference, I bring my knowledge of my paralyzed body. Together we analyze what is wrong, what treatment is advisable and what its impact is likely to be-on the problem and on my ability to function independently.

—Hugh Gallagher, Black Bird Fly Away[23]

Diagnostic testing, including sleep studies, blood work, and tests for other illness, is critical to determine if other medical interventions are warranted for individuals with PPS. When medical interventions are ruled out or exhausted, managing fatigue involves education and implementing strategies to manage fatigue.[11,24,25]

Currently, treatment of managing fatigue with individuals with PPS is focused on symptom management and individual strategies, such as energy conservation, pacing techniques, lifestyle modifications, and work simplification.[25-29] Additional high-quality research is needed in the areas of energy conservation and pacing interventions for PPS-related fatigue.[24]

Pacing and energy conservation techniques are common strategies used to address fatigue in other chronic health conditions. Matuska and colleagues[30] reported individuals with multiple sclerosis participating in a 6-week energy conservation course reported that strategies were effective in managing fatigue. Van Heest and colleagues[31] reported reduction in fatigue, an increase in self-efficacy, and higher quality of life in participants in a one-to-one fatigue management course for persons with chronic fatigue and pain. A systematic review on the effectiveness of pacing with chronic pain did not impact pain severity; however, there was evidence pacing "can assist in reducing the interference of fatigue, joint stiffness and decrease physical activity variability."[32]

Fatigue is a subjective experience and can be difficult to define for individuals with PPS. Choosing a reliable and accurate scale that is easy to use and valid for persons with PPS provides a picture of how fatigue impacts daily life and drives intervention.[33] Using a journal and writing a daily activity log is a useful tool for the polio survivor to understand the impact of their activity expenditure and how it may correlate with their fatigue, pain, and weakness. A daily activity log can be quite informative and provides useful insight into the activities in which the polio survivor is engaging daily.[25,27]

Grace Young,[28] an occupational therapist and polio survivor, developed an energy conservation program for individuals with PPS that includes the pathophysiology of polio. She writes, "If the polio survivor does not understand his or her disorder, it is very difficult to implement necessary intervention and strategies."

Specific energy conservation techniques should be tailored to the polio survivor's life. Understanding life roles, values, and goals is necessary to help facilitate and support the individual. The goal is to promote strategies to adapt rather than to take away or stop.[34]

At the height of the epidemic between 1950 and 1954, polio affected 22,000 US citizens each year.[35] Many of these individuals with PPS are aging; therefore, participating in leisure activities may be affected by fatigue and weakness. Walking on the beach or playing a round of golf may no longer be possible. Cook and colleagues[34] concluded that people with disabilities do not reap the "retirement benefit," and fatigue may not change for the better but get worse as people with disabilities "age into retirement." Managing fatigue for individuals with PPS becomes more crucial with aging because of the potential negative impact on quality of life.

Hugh Gallagher,[23] a noted scholar and expert on Franklin D. Roosevelt and himself a polio survivor, explains in his autobiography, *Black Bird Fly Away*, "My muscle power *and endurance are as coins in my purse. I only have so many and they will only buy so much. I must live within my means and to do this I have to economize: what do I want to buy and how can I buy it for the least possible cost?"* [23]

This is a powerful analogy for the polio survivor. Describing the energy budget as coins in a purse quantifies the energy level. Individuals with PPS can be more judicious about how they spend their energy. It is the beginning of self-reflection, understanding how energy conservation and pacing techniques can alleviate the symptoms of fatigue, pain, and weakness.

Using technology, such as smart watches, smart phones, mobile apps, and smart home devices, assists the individual with PPS to manage their output of energy. Smart watches can track steps to avoid overuse, and smart home devices can turn on lights, open shades, and manage garage doors, allowing for more efficient use of movement while in the home. Equipment, such as comfort height toilets, shower chairs, and handheld showers, are not only recommended for safety but also reduce the load on already weakened polio muscles.

Stair lifts, or electric chair lifts, provide much needed rest for fatiguing muscles. Ergonomic set up of the home and work area allows muscles affected by polio to be more efficient. Ten Katen and colleagues[36] reported that decreasing physical demands and using ergonomic changes in the workplace allowed polio survivors to maintain their work activities. Other lifestyle modifications include smoking cessation and weight loss. Weight gain is a common complaint among individuals with PPS; consulting with a nutritionist should be considered.[27]

Assistive Devices

The use of mobility aids for locomotion is shown to reduce self-reported levels of fatigue.[3,4,24,37] Assistive devices, such as canes, forearm crutches, rolling walkers, and 4-wheeled rolling walkers, may be beneficial. It is important to consider the individual's strengths, weaknesses, and compensations during gait to identify the best possible device. The device should be lightweight and ergonomic. An opportunity to trial device options with patients is recommended to ensure proper fit, function, and safety. For example, with left lower-extremity weakness, use of a cane in the right hand would be recommended. If there is weakness in the right upper extremity, a cane may not be the best choice. When adding an assistive device, the whole patient must be considered to avoid causing any new problems.[24]

Wheelchairs and Scooters

Wheelchairs and scooters may also enhance quality of life and reduce fatigue. When choosing a wheelchair, many factors must be considered. These factors include the impairments, desired activities/participation, environment (work and home), the ability to transport the chair, and support. For example, when an individual has marked upper-extremity weakness, a manual wheelchair or scooter may not be recommended because of concern for additional upper-extremity overuse. Use of the upper extremities is the key to an individual with PPS's independence and must be preserved. In this case, a power wheelchair may be recommended if the environment is suitable.[3,24]

Orthotic Intervention

Orthotic interventions may be beneficial to improve ambulation in certain individuals with PPS. The energy cost of walking was found to be 40% higher in individuals with PPS as compared with healthy subjects.[38] The use of orthoses has been shown to improve walking efficiency. When choosing a device, it is important to respect the individual's existing compensations. A comprehensive examination is needed to identify impairments, such as muscle performance, joint integrity, pain, fatigue, and range of motion. The orthosis prescription should be a multidisciplinary process that also considers fall history, individual goals, lifestyle, and degree of brace acceptance. Biomechanical analysis of ambulation pattern may also assist in optimal design and function of the orthosis.[39] Overcorrecting compensations with an orthosis may lead to a decline in walking efficiency and would not be tolerated. Lightweight materials, such as carbon fiber or carbon fiber–reinforced plastic, have been shown to improve walking efficiency as compared with plastic, metal, and leather.[24,39] Kelley and DiBello[40] developed a classification system to assist health care providers in the clinical decision-making process involved in orthotic prescription for individuals with PPS. Identifying the optimal brace is necessary to improve fatigue and quality of life.

Exercise

Individuals with fatigue and PPS often work to their maximum ability, which leads to muscle overuse. This occurrence is termed low-frequency fatigue and refers to fatigue that persists for long periods of time before ability returns. This low-frequency fatigue may last for hours, days, or months depending on the intensity and duration of the associated activity.[37]

Research on exercise training is limited. Koopman[41] reported that muscle strengthening and aerobic exercise may be beneficial and increase functional capacity in individuals with PPS. Physically active individuals with PPS were found to have fewer symptoms and higher functional levels than those that were inactive.[42] Pacing, rest intervals, and weight loss related to exercise is recommended.[41] A recent study by Voorn and colleagues[43] found that severely fatigued individuals with PPS were not able to adhere to a high-intensity 4-month home-based exercise program. There was no improvement in cardiorespiratory fitness, muscle function, or aerobic capacity. Given the heterogeneity of this population, exercise should be tailored to the individual by a health care professional familiar with PPS to prescribe an appropriate exercise program to avoid fatigue[43] (**Box 4**).

Case Study

Mr W is a 62-year-old man who contracted bulbar and paralytic polio at age 5, which affected his breathing and bilateral lower-extremity strength. His history included several days in an iron lung, multiple surgeries related to polio, and use of bilateral lower-extremity braces until age 12. Chief complaints consisted of severe fatigue, lower-extremity weakness and atrophy, and low-back and bilateral lower-extremity pain (7/10 at worst on 0–10 Numerical Pain Rating Scale). Mr W described feeling a "mental and physical shut down" that interfered with his ability to work, exercise, perform activities of daily living (ADLs), do yard work, and participate in outdoor leisure activities. These symptoms intensified gradually over a 10-year period, which led him to seek care at a multidisciplinary postpolio clinic in 2015.

During the initial multidisciplinary examination (physiatrist, physical therapist, and occupational therapist), Mr W was tearful as he described his history and current symptoms. In his role as a manager, he was required to walk and stand for up to 10 hours per day, which included a large retail space and stairs to a second-floor office. He lived with his wife in a 2-level home (15–20 steps inside) with the bedroom and full bathroom on the second floor. Avocational interests consisted of kayaking, reading, and watching movies. Mr W went to the gym 4 to 5 days per week for a total of 1.5 hours per session. His exercise program included 30 minutes of swimming laps, intensive upper-extremity weights, and 30 to 45 minutes on the treadmill.

Box 4
Talking points for conserving energy

Home modifications
- Install comfort height or handicapped toilet
- Use a shower chair
- Install grab bars in bathroom
- Increase height of any seating in the home
- Avoid stairs, consider 1-floor living
- Install stair lift if consistently using stairs

Car and driving adaptations
- Obtain handicapped placard or handicapped plate
- Change gas pedal to left side if right leg is weak
- Consider hand controls if both legs affected by old polio
- Use cruise control when possible

Community mobility
- Use mobility aids to prevent overuse
- Park close to store entrances
- Identify a place to take a rest break if needed
- Shop online to avoid waiting in lines or shop on off hours

Time management
- Organize day around time of optimal energy
- Prioritize and plan activities ahead of time

Assistive devices and power mobility for locomotion efficiency
- Use prescribed assistive device
- Consider use of power wheelchair or scooter

Brace management
- Collaborate with orthotist and physical therapist for optimal lower-extremity bracing options

Exercise recommendations
- Educate patient in nonfatiguing patient-specific exercise program
- Consider use of smart devices to identify optimal steps or distance per day

Sleep
- Consider steep study
- Educate about sleep hygiene
- Recommend short, frequent rest periods with nap as needed

Assistive technology
- Home and work automation systems for environmental control, including smart phone apps
- Recommend assistive technology evaluation by experts

Work simplification and ergonomic setup
- Create a work triangle with primary project in the center and supplies at sides
- Use supportive chair and footrest
- Place monitor arm's length away and use mouse and external keyboard with laptops

Adapted from Cole MH, Ryan LA. Energy Conservation and Pacing. In: Silver JK, Gawne AC, eds. Postpolio Syndrome. Philadelphia, PA: Hanley & Belfus; 2004:261-273.

Mr W reported no significant past medical history except for high blood pressure and poliomyelitis. His medications included amlodipine, lisinopril, alprazolam, and hydrocodone. He reported 3 falls in the prior year and 1 to 2 near falls per month. He woke twice per night because of pain and periodic limb movements.

Mr W was independent with all functional mobility, including ADLs, bed mobility, transfers, and ambulation. He ambulated without an assistive device or brace with a walking speed of 0.82 m per second.

Examination of strength using manual muscle testing (MMT)[44,45] revealed upper-extremity strength of 4–/5 to 4/5 bilaterally with the left side slightly weaker. Left lower-extremity strength was 3 to 3+/5 throughout, except the ankle at 2/5. Right (R) lower-extremity MMT was 3/5 throughout, except hip extension and knee flexion 2/5 and ankle 1/5. Lower-extremity strength testing revealed muscle fasciculations and jerky movement. Atrophy was present in the R lower extremity.

The FSS score was 63/63 with a mean score 7, signifying the highest possible level of fatigue. The initial 3-day log revealed increased pain and fatigue with all work and leisure activities. Mr W made multiple trips between the upstairs office and retail floor with complaints of lower-extremity weakness and pain. Although he enjoyed going the gym, he reported fatigue and muscle weakness in upper and lower extremities for several hours afterward (**Box 5**).

At first follow-up in 2016:

- FSS remained unchanged.
- Mr W stopped working and applied for Social Security Disability Insurance.
- Mr W began using a right foot brace intermittently (foot up or posterior leaf spring ankle foot orthosis [PLS-AFO]).
- Mr W added an arm ergometer without decreasing other exercises.
- Mr W declined a sleep study despite reports of periodic limb movement.
- Mr W declined speaking with a mental health provider.
- Mr W reported "life is good."

At second follow-up visit in 2017:

- Mr W moved to a 1-level condominium with an elevator.
- Mr W reported less pain and fatigue when using energy conservation and pacing techniques.

Box 5
Plan of care

1. Additional medical work-up
   a. MRI lumbar spine to rule out other causes of weakness and pain
   b. Referral for sleep study (leg jumping, fatigue)
   c. Bone mineral density testing
   d. Additional laboratory work

2. Referral to brace clinic

3. Energy conservation and pacing
   a. Reduce stair use—consider stair chair lift
   b. Use R foot up brace or PLS-AFO for increased gait efficiency
   c. Reduce exercise intensity and frequency using PPS exercise guideline recommendations
   d. Lifestyle and workplace modifications:
      i. Decrease standing and frequency of stair climbing at work
      ii. Decrease work overtime hours
      iii. Consider applying for long-term disability

4. Referral to mental health provider
   a. Rehabilitation psychologist

5. Patient education
   a. Fall risk reduction
   b. Trial assistive devices
   c. Home modifications/adaptive equipment, including installing a comfort height toilet, increase height of all seating

- Mr W participated in leisure activities, including gardening and kayaking.
- Mr W used a straight cane for community ambulation.
- Mr W improved FSS to 51/63, a mean score of 5.6.
- Mr W improved walking speed to 1.16 m/s with an R PLS-AFO.
- Exercise program was modified based on the recommended postpolio exercise guidelines (**Table 1**).

A multidisciplinary team approach is necessary to address fatigue in individuals with polio. Occupational and physical therapists use energy conservation and pacing techniques in their practice and provide a comprehensive approach in addressing individuals with PPS. Input from a multidisciplinary team, including physical therapist, occupational therapist, speech and language pathologist, nutritionist, psychologist, orthotist, and physician, is needed to address the multifactorial issues related to PPS and fatigue.[11]

FUTURE DIRECTIONS
Intravenous Immunoglobulin

PPS is a progressive disorder characterized by general and muscular fatigue, new muscle weakness and atrophy, pain, and loss of function. The cause, although not fully understood, is thought to be multifactorial. The pathogenesis includes ongoing scattered motor neuron loss, denervation of enlarged motor units and increased expression of several inflammatory cytokines in the cerebral spinal fluid.[11] This inflammatory process in the CNS is thought to contribute to PPS symptoms of fatigue, pain, and muscle weakness. There is evidence that intravenous immunoglobulin (IVIg) may benefit some individuals with PPS.[3,11,46]

In 2015, Östlund and colleagues[46] identified responders to IVIg as those individuals with PPS with high levels of fatigue and/or pain (scoring 20 or higher on the VAS), muscle weakness and atrophy in the lower extremities, and reduced physical function. Responders had a positive response with vitality and/or bodily pain on the Short Form-36 (SF-36). Nonresponders were identified as having lower level of fatigue and pain, good mental health, and good physical function.

Previous studies offer evidence that treatment with IVIg provides some benefit to individuals with PPS. Different methodology and outcome measures, however, limit interpretation of the results. In 2016, Camprubi[47] described the ongoing FORCE: Efficacy-Safety of Intravenous Immunoglobulins in PPS, which is a multicenter

Table 1
Case outcomes

	Initial Evaluation 2015	First Yearly Follow-Up 2016	Second Yearly Follow-Up 2017 (Moved to Maine, 1-Level Home with Elevator)
FSS	63/63 or mean 7	63/63 or mean 7	51/63 or mean 5.6
Activities balance; confidence scale, %	63.75	59.3	75
Gait speed (self-selected)	0.82 m/s without brace	1.05 m/s R foot up	1.16 m/s R AFO brace
Falls	4–6 in prior year	1–3 in prior year	1–3 in prior year
Pain (0–10 Numerical Pain Rating Scale)	7/10 at worst	5/10 at worst	4/10 at worst

prospective randomized placebo-controlled, double blind study to assess for optimal dosing estimated to end in 2020.

Although there is limited evidence that IVIg impacts fatigue thus far, the presence of fatigue appears to be a qualifying factor for responders of IVIg intervention.[46] Additional research studies on IVIg and other pharmacologic interventions and its impact on fatigue for individuals with PPS are needed.

SUMMARY

Individuals living with PPS face many restrictions in activity and participation in different aspects of their life. Fatigue is one of the most disabling complaints of individuals with PPS. In essence, their world shrinks. Fatigue is often referred to as the invisible disability. PPS is diagnosed by exclusion; therefore, a thorough medical workup is needed to rule out all other causes of fatigue based on the MoD criteria for PPS.[3,5] A sleep study should be considered for individuals with PPS. Use of self-reported outcome measures of fatigue are sensitive and reliable, but some lack the ability to detect change over time. Although fatigue is cited frequently in the literature, there are few high-quality studies supporting the effectiveness of energy conservation and pacing. Despite the lack of strong evidence, energy conservation and pacing are hallmark strategies to address fatigue in PPS. In addition, lifestyle changes, assistive devices, wheelchairs, power mobility, and bracing may aid in reducing fatigue in individuals with PPS to allow for increased participation in meaningful activities.

There are many different definitions of fatigue, energy conservation, and pacing in the literature. Establishing a definition by consensus for individuals with PPS would greatly enhance research. Measurement of fatigue should be examined further using World Health Organization (WHO) International Classifications of Functioning, Disability and Health (ICF) Model to foster a common language.

I have learned that, however impressive a recovery you make, you don't 'conquer' or 'overcome' polio in any meaningful sense, you merely adapt to the limitations it imposes and—-if you are fortunate—discover within yourself resources you might not otherwise have found.
—Tony Gould, author of A Summer Plague: Polio and Its Survivors[48]

CLINICS CARE POINTS

- Fatigue, a common complaint in individuals with postpolio syndrome, is defined as an overwhelming sustained feeling of exhaustion and diminished capacity for physical and mental work.[7]

- A comprehensive medical work-up is indicated to rule out all other causes of fatigue.[11]

- A sleep study should be considered for individuals with postpolio syndrome and fatigue.[6,49]

- Self-reported outcome measures, such as the Fatigue Severity Scale, are reliable and valid tools to measure fatigue.[17,20]

- Individualized energy conservation and pacing techniques are commonly used interventions for reducing fatigue.[11,24]

- Assistive devices, wheelchairs, power mobility, and bracing may aid in reducing fatigue in individuals with postpolio syndrome.[24,37]

- A multidisciplinary approach to fatigue is necessary to enhance quality of life.[11,24]

DISCLOSURE

The authors have nothing to disclose.

REFERENCES

1. Post-Polio Syndrome Fact Sheet. National Institute of Neurological Disorders and Stroke. 2020. Available at: https://www.ninds.nih.gov/Disorders/Patient-Caregiver-Education/Fact-Sheets/Post-Polio-Syndrome-Fact-Sheet. Accessed August 2, 2020.
2. Abdulraheem IS, Saka MJ, Saka AO. Postpolio syndrome: epidemiology, pathogenesis and management. J Infect Dis Immun 2011;3(15):247–57.
3. Farbu E. Update on current and emerging treatment options for post-polio syndrome. Ther Clin Risk Manag 2010;2010(default):307–13.
4. Farbu E, Gilhus NE, Barnes MP, et al. EFNS guideline on diagnosis and management of post-polio syndrome. Report of an EFNS Task Force. Eur J Neurol 2006; 13(8):795–801.
5. March of Dimes International Conference on Post-Polio Syndrome Identifying Best Practices in Diagnosis & Care. 2000. Available at: https://www.polioplace.org/sites/default/files/files/MOD-%20Identifying.pdf. Accessed August 2, 2020.
6. Tersteeg I. Fatigue in patients with post-polio syndrome is determined by physical as well as psychological factors. J Rehabil Med Stiftelsen Rehabiliteringsinformation 2011; (49Supple):42-42.
7. Taber's Online. Available at: https://www.tabers.com/tabersonline/view/Tabers-Dictionary/757231/all/fatigue. Accessed June 15, 2020.
8. Smith HS. Handbook of fatigue in health and disease. New York: Nova Science Publishers, Inc; 2011. Available at: https://login.treadwell.idm.oclc.org/login?url=https://search.ebscohost.com/login.aspx?
direct=true&db=nlebk&AN=382380&site=eds-live&
scope=site.
9. Östlund G, Wahlin Å, Sunnerhagen KS, et al. Post polio syndrome: fatigued patients a specific subgroup? J Rehabil Med 2011;43(1):39–45.
10. Bruno RL, Cohen JM, Galski T, et al. The neuroanatomy of post-polio fatigue. Arch Phys Med Rehabil 1994;75(5):498–504.
11. Shing S, Chipika R, Finegan E, et al. Post-polio syndrome: more than just a lower motor neuron disease. Front Neurol 2019;10. https://doi.org/10.3389/fneur.2019.00773.
12. Viana C, Pradella-Hallinan M, Quadros A, et al. Circadian variation of fatigue in both patients with paralytic poliomyelitis and post-polio syndrome. Arq Neuropsiquiatr 2013;71(7):442–5.
13. eRomigi A, eMaestri M. Circadian fatigue or unrecognized restless legs syndrome? The post-polio syndrome model. Front Neurol 2014;5. https://doi.org/10.3389/fneur.2014.00115.
14. Léotard A, Lévy J, Hartley S, et al. Sleep disorders in aging polio survivors: a systematic review. Ann Phys Rehabil Med 2019;63(6):543–53. Available at: https://login.treadwell.idm.oclc.org/login?url=https://search.ebscohost.com/login.aspx?
direct=true&db=edselp&AN=S1877065719301800&site=eds-live&scope=site.
15. Moses S. Fatigue. Family practice notebook. Available at: https://fpnotebook.com/Rheum/Sx/Ftg.htm. Accessed August 9, 2020.
16. Jensen MP, Alschuler KN, Smith AE, et al. Pain and fatigue in persons with post-polio syndrome: independent effects on functioning. Arch Phys Med Rehabil 2011;92(11):1796–801.

17. Vasconcelos JOM, Prokhorenko OA, Kelley KF, et al. A comparison of fatigue scales in postpoliomyelitis syndrome. Arch Phys Med Rehabil 2006;87(9): 1213–7.
18. Koopman FS, Brehm MA, Heerkens YF, et al. Measuring fatigue in polio survivors: content comparison and reliability of the Fatigue Severity Scale and the Checklist Individual Strength. J Rehabil Med 2014;46(8):761–7.
19. On AY, Oncu J, Atamaz F, et al. Impact of post-polio-related fatigue on quality of life. J Rehabil Med 2006;38(5):329–32.
20. Horemans HL, Nollet F, Beelen A, et al. A comparison of 4 questionnaires to measure fatigue in postpoliomyelitis syndrome. Arch Phys Med Rehabil 2004;85(3): 392–8.
21. Krupp LB, LaRocca NG, Muir-Nash J, et al. The fatigue severity scale. Application to patients with multiple sclerosis and systemic lupus erythematosus. Arch Neurol 1989;46(10):1121–3.
22. Valko PO, Bassetti CL, Bloch KE, et al. Validation of the fatigue severity scale in a Swiss cohort. Sleep 2008;31(11):1601–7.
23. Gallagher H. Black bird fly away. Arlington, (VA): Vandamere Press; 1988.
24. Lo JK, Robinson LR. Post-polio syndrome and the late effects of poliomyelitis: part 2. treatment, management, and prognosis. Muscle Nerve 2018;58(6):760–9.
25. Silver JK, Gawne AC. Postpolio syndrome. Hanley & Belfus: An Affiliate of Elsevier; 2004.
26. Trojan DA, Finch L. Management of post-polio syndrome. Neurorehabilitation 1997;8(2):93–105.
27. Silver J. Post-polio: a guide for polio survivors & their families. New Haven: Yale University Press; 2001.
28. Young GR. Occupational therapy and the postpolio syndrome. Am J Occup Ther 1989;43(2):97–103.
29. Jubelt B, Agre JC. Characteristics and management of postpolio syndrome. JAMA 2000;284(4):412–4.
30. Matuska K, Mathiowetz V, Finlayson M. Use and perceived effectiveness of energy conservation strategies for managing multiple sclerosis fatigue. Am J Occup Ther 2007;61(1):62–9.
31. Van Heest KNL, Mogush AR, Mathiowetz VG. Effects of a one-to-one fatigue management course for people with chronic conditions and fatigue. Am J Occup Ther 2017;71(4):1–9.
32. Guy L, McKinstry C, Bruce C. Effectiveness of pacing as a learned strategy for people with chronic pain: a systematic review. Am J Occup Ther 2019; 73(3):1–10.
33. Whitehead L. The measurement of fatigue in chronic illness: a systematic review of unidimensional and multidimensional fatigue measures. J Pain Symptom Manage 2009;37(1):107–28.
34. Cook KF, Molton IR, Jensen MP. Fatigue and aging with a disability. Arch Phys Med Rehabil 2011;92(7):1126–33.
35. Trevelyan B, Smallman-Raynor M, Cliff A. The spatial dynamics of poliomyelitis in the United States: from epidemic emergence to vaccine-induced retreat, 1910-1971. Ann Assoc Am Geogr 2005;95(2):269.
36. Ten Katen K, Beelen A, Nollet F, et al. Overcoming barriers to work participation for patients with postpoliomyelitis syndrome. Disabil Rehabil 2011;33(6):522–9.
37. Silva IST, Sunnerhagen KS, Willén C, et al. The extent of using mobility assistive devices can partly explain fatigue among persons with late effects of polio - a retrospective registry study in Sweden. BMC Neurol 2016;16:1–6.

38. Brehm M-A, Nollet F, Harlaar J. Energy demands of walking in persons with post-poliomyelitis syndrome: relationship with muscle strength and reproducibility. Arch Phys Med Rehabil 2006;87(1):136–40.
39. Brehm MA, Beelen A, Doorenbosch CA, et al. Effect of carbon-composite knee-ankle-foot orthoses on walking efficiency and gait in former polio patients. J Rehabil Med Stiftelsen Rehabiliteringsinformation 2007;39(8):651–7.
40. Kelley C, DiBello TV. Orthotic assessment for individuals with postpolio syndrome: a classification system. J Prosthet Orthot 2007;19(4):109–13.
41. Koopman FS. Treatment for postpolio syndrome. Gilhus NE, de Visser M, eds Cochrane Database Syst Rev. (5). Available at: https://login.treadwell.idm.oclc.org/login?url=https://search.ebscohost.com/login.aspx?direct=true&db=edschh&AN=edschh.CD007818&site=eds-live&scope=site. Accessed August 13, 2020.
42. Rekand T, Korv J, Farbu E, et al. Lifestyle and late effects after poliomyelitis. A risk factor study of two populations. Acta Neurol Scand 2004;109(2):120–5.
43. Voorn EL, Koopman FS, Brehm MA, et al. Aerobic exercise training in post-polio syndrome: process evaluation of a randomized controlled trial. PLoS One 2016;11(7):e0159280.
44. Hislop HH, Avers D, Borwn M. Daniels's and Worthington's muscle testing. St Louis (MO): Saunders; 2014.
45. Medical Research Council. Aids to the examination of the peripheral nervous system: Memorandum No. 45. Available at: https://mrc.ukri.org/research/facilities-and-resources-for-researchers/mrc-scales/mrc-muscle-scale/. Accessed September 15, 2008.
46. Östlund G, Broman L, Werhagen L, et al. Immunoglobulin treatment in post-polio syndrome: identification of responders and non-responders. J Rehabil Med 2015;47(8):727–33.
47. Camprubi S. FORCE: EFFICACY-SAFETY OF INTRAVENOUS IMMUNOGLOBULIN IN PPS...1st Australasia-Pacific Post-Polio Conference: Polio - Life Stage Matters. Sydney, Australia 20-22 September 2016. J Rehabil Med Stiftelsen Rehabiliteringsinformation 2016;48(8):754.
48. Gould T. A summer plague: polio and its survivors. New Haven: Yale University Press; 1995.
49. Silver J, Aiello D. What internists need to know about postpolio syndrome. Cleve Clin J Med 2002;69:704–6, 709.

Bracing
Upper and Lower Limb Orthoses

Claudia A. Wheeler, DO

KEYWORDS

- AFO (ankle-foot orthosis) • DMU (double metal upright)
- KAFO (knee-ankle-foot orthosis) • Wrist-hand orthosis) • Stance-control knee
- Rocker bottom shoe • Leg length discrepancy

KEY POINTS

- Goals of bracing in polio and postpolio: prevent deformity, optimize joint mechanics, and support weakened muscles by promoting an energy-efficient gait pattern that reduces compensatory mechanisms.
- Risk of falls/injury in polio survivors: the risk of falls and injury caused by falls is increased in polio survivors. Compliance with bracing can help reduce risk of falls.
- Polio-specific considerations to improve compliance: energy conservation, weight of device, body mechanics, and unique anatomic considerations.
- Best practices: selection of best candidates, use of outcome measures to measure efficacy, and consideration of energy conservation in brace design.

DISCUSSION
Goals of Bracing in Polio and Postpolio Syndrome

In the acute polio phase, the goal of bracing is to prevent deformity and to support functional gait by assisting weakened muscles. The most common gait deviations in the acute phase that need orthotic management are flaccid foot drop during swing phase and steppage gait pattern.

In children with acute polio, preventing a rigid equinovarus deformity is key to a successful tendon transfer surgery once skeletally mature.[1] In the residual poliomyelitis paralysis phase, the goal is to optimize joint mechanics and support weakened muscles by promoting an energy-efficient gait pattern that reduces compensatory mechanisms.

Principles of Bracing in Polio and Postpolio Syndrome

The basic principles of bracing in the polio population are based on energy conservation and preventing deformity or skin breakdown.

LPG Physiatry, 765 Allens Avenue, Suite 110, Providence, RI 02905, USA
E-mail address: claudia.wheeler@lifespan.org

Phys Med Rehabil Clin N Am 32 (2021) 509–526
https://doi.org/10.1016/j.pmr.2021.03.001
1047-9651/21/© 2021 Elsevier Inc. All rights reserved.

o Leave as many joints free (unlocked) as possible.[1-3]
o Energy consumption increases with locked joints.[1-3]
o Make the orthosis as lightweight as possible. Thermoplastics and carbon fiber are lighter than metal and leather.[3]
o Maximize total contact and reduce pressure over bony prominences. Because polio causes muscle atrophy, there is less soft tissue muscle mass. Point pressure over a bony prominence could lead to skin breakdown.[3]
o Braces can provide support, relieve pain, and correct a flexible deformity.[4]
o In the case of fixed deformity, it is best to try to correct or reduce it surgically or with aggressive therapy before applying a brace.[4]
o In children, attempt to discontinue the orthosis at time of skeletal maturity when surgical stabilization can be done, if appropriate.[1]

Extent of Bracing

The extent of bracing depends on the muscle power about the hip, knee, and ankle joints. If quadriceps muscle strength is greater than or equal to 3, bracing need not extend above the knee unless there is ligamentous damage or knee hyperextension.[1] In the case of knee hyperextension with sufficient quadriceps strength, a knee-ankle-foot orthosis (KAFO) may be needed to prevent further knee deformity and reduce gait deviation.[1,5] It is recommended that bracing be based on individual assessment and evaluation. It is common for polio survivors to have a leg length discrepancy, and this should be assessed for and measured. Application of a lift inside or outside the shoe as necessary should be used for correction of up to 75% of the leg length discrepancy. The shoe is an extension of the brace and should be addressed for smooth rollover into stance phase. A rocker sole eases the transition from midstance to toe-off, and a rocker heel transitions from initial contact to loading phase. Patients with hip extensor weakness should be carefully evaluated for appropriateness of a rocker bottom sole because it may produce some additional knee instability through stance.[5]

BRACING EVALUATION

- Detailed history: medical comorbidities, falls, degree of independence with mobility-related activities of daily living.
- Secondary conditions associated with postpolio include, but are not limited to, fatigue, pain, respiratory complaints, depression, sleep disorder, falls, bone and joint disorders, impaired cardiovascular function, diabetes, bladder dysfunction, and skin problems.[6]
- Physical examination: oxygen saturation, pulse; assess for asymmetry, joint deformity, range of motion (ROM), strength, gait for ambulatory patients, and functional mobility:
  o Bed mobility
  o Rolling
  o Sit to stand
  o Transfers
  o Stairs
  o Wheelchair mobility if appropriate
- Assessing the patient's goals and feasibility of an orthosis achieving those goals.
- Discussion about optimal assistive device to allow optimally energy-efficient, safe mobility on various terrains and environmental obstacles, such as stairs and ramps.

- Discussion about reasonable expectations and the path to achieving those expectations includes a commitment to compliance with the device and gait training for optimal use.
- Although bracing joints may provide improved stability with some activities (eg, walking), the device may alter other functional activities (eg, transfers, stairs, driving) and cosmesis.
- Discussion about the risks of not using an orthotic device and long-term sequelae of impaired joint mechanics and compensatory strategies.
- Best outcomes are achieved with joint decision making at a multidisciplinary bracing clinic with input from physiatrist, orthotist, physical or occupational therapist, and the patient/patient's caregivers/staff.

Orthotic Devices/Materials/Joints

Ankle-foot orthoses
The ankle-foot orthosis (AFO) provides multidirectional joint stability and protection by assisting clearance during swing phase and stabilization in stance phase. The angle of the ankle affects the kinematics of the knee. The type of material, stiffness, and trim lines affect the stability provided, allowing customization to meet the patient's individual needs.[5]

Posterior leaf spring
The posterior leaf spring (PLS) AFO provides foot clearance during swing phase and minimal control of ankle eversion or inversion (**Fig. 1**). It can slow ankle plantar flexion, which prevents foot slap. The PLS AFO is lightweight and is best suited for patients with minimal weakness in the ankle dorsiflexor muscle.[5]

Solid ankle
The solid ankle AFO provides significant ankle and foot control in multiple planes during stance phase (**Fig. 2**). It is bulkier and more rigid in design than the PLS AFO. This design may benefit patients with painful ankles because it can completely limit motion. Pairing a solid ankle AFO with a rocker bottom shoe can assist in transition through stance phase.[5]

Articulated ankle
The articulated ankle AFO is a solid AFO with an articulated ankle joint to provide a predetermined amount of ROM through the anatomic ankle (**Figs. 3** and **4**). The amount of dorsiflexion and plantarflexion can be individually determined and should match the anatomic ROM available at the patient's ankle. The articulated ankle AFO can provide more than adequate plantarflexion control; however, dorsiflexion control is more difficult because of the mechanical stresses on the fabrication material. This type of AFO is used for lightweight or limited-ambulation populations. A community ambulator would be best served by a double-action or triple-action ankle joint, generally used in metal upright AFOs.[5] For average postpolio patients with calf and thigh weakness, the most satisfactory below-knee brace is hinged and allows free plantar flexion of 15° to 20° while permitting only 5° to 10° of ankle dorsiflexion. This brace allows stability buy enough ankle mobility to facilitate stair walking.[4]

Ground reaction
The ground-reaction AFO provides stability in the knee during stance through a posterior ground-reaction force that blocks forward tibial progression. Ground reaction can be achieved through a full-length foot plate and, if needed, an anterior shell. Prefabricated ground-reaction AFOs are also available for patients without significant

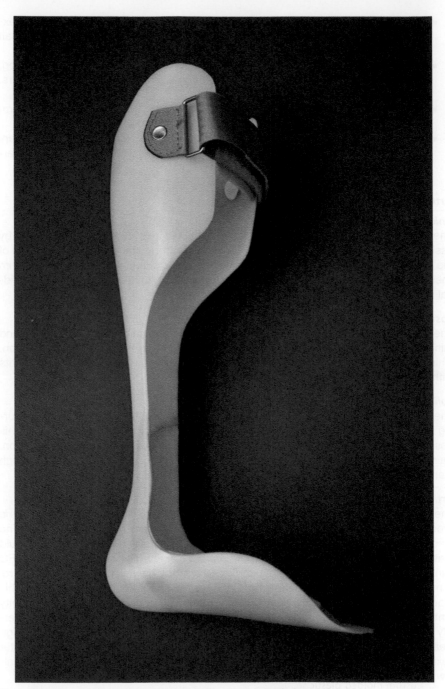

Fig. 1. Custom molded plastic PLS AFO with sulcus length foot plate.

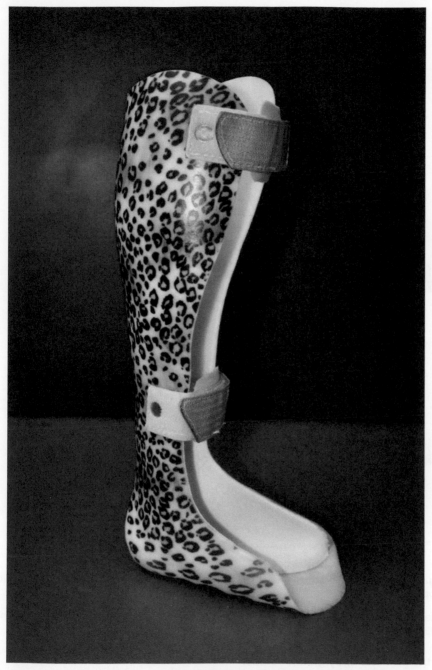

Fig. 2. Custom molded plastic semisolid ankle AFO with three-quarter length foot plate.

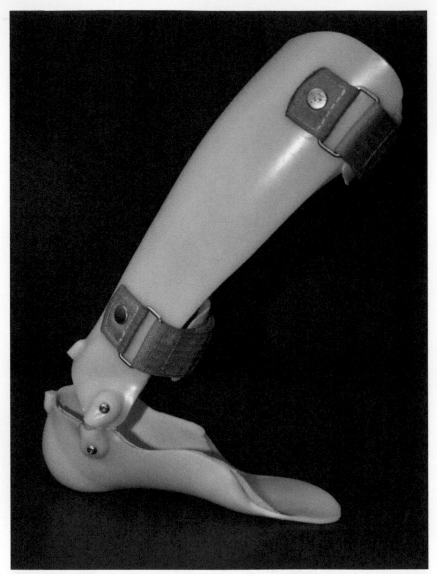

Fig. 3. Custom molded articulated ankle AFO with dorsiflexion assist and plantar flexion stop.

anatomic deformity that can achieve subtalar neutral because these braces are not adjustable.[5]

Articulated rear-entry ground reaction
Articulated rear-entry ground-reaction AFOs provide numerous benefits to the polio population requiring knee and ankle stability. The anterior lower leg stop provides resistance during stance with adjustable dorsiflexion and plantar flexion stops as well as a possible dorsiflexion assist to allow improved clearance with swing and a smooth transition during stance. This design can be beneficial in polio survivors with balance impairment in need of energy conservation.[5]

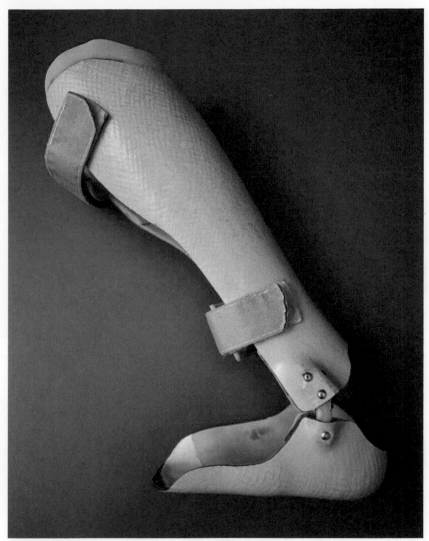

Fig. 4. Custom molded carbon fiber articulated ankle AFO with dorsiflexion assist and adjustable ankle joints.

Dorsiflexion restricting
In polio survivors with calf muscle weakness (gastrocnemius-soleus complex), dorsiflexion-restricting AFOs increase forward progression of center of pressure in midstance and reduce ankle dorsiflexion and knee flexion in midstance and terminal stance.[7]

Double metal upright
The double metal upright (DMU) AFO is an older design that is still used for patients with significant fluctuating edema or who are not willing to change design (**Fig. 5**). Ankle varus or valgus correction with this style is achieved with use of a T strap. The uprights are attached to the shoe, which limits the patient's shoe wear choices.

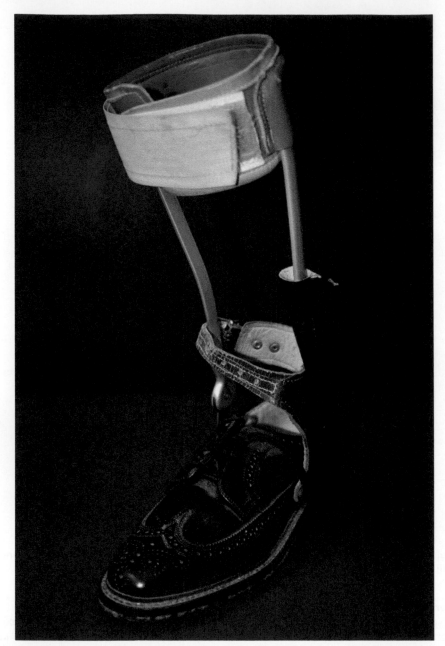

Fig. 5. Conventional DMU dorsiflexion-assist AFO with single-action ankle and ankle varus control T strap.

Double-action ankle joints are used on both sides. In the anterior compartment, a pin is used to control tibial advancement in stance for a knee extension moment at heel-off. Springs are not generally used in the anterior compartment because they do not provide enough resistance to dorsiflexion in loading given the patient's body weight.

In the posterior compartment, either a spring or pin is effective to aid in foot clearance in swing phase. The spring is preferred when limiting plantar flexion for limb stabilization during stance is not needed because it smooths the transition through initial contact to loading. Historically, Klenzak joints with dorsiflexion assist at the ankle were used for patients with polio. This traditional design allows clearance during swing but does not provide resistance to tibial progression in stance. It was noted that, over time, patients wearing this design developed plantar flexor weakness and lost their stance control, which results in overuse of the contralateral side. The Klenzak joint should be reserved for patients with strong ankle plantar flexors.[5]

Knee-ankle-foot orthoses

The KAFO extends proximally above the knee for patients requiring more stability at the knee because of hyperextension moment or knee buckling because of quadriceps muscle weakness. In the polio and postpolio populations, using a KAFO with ischial containment or quadrilateral thigh portion design can support weight bearing through the weak limb to reduce contralateral limb stress. This design is particularly helpful in patients with fatigue, contralateral pain, or contralateral weakness, allowing increased time in stance on the limb wearing the KAFO.[5]

Knee Joints

Posterior offset

The posterior offset knee joint is ideal for patients with unilateral genu recurvatum, or hyperextension at the knee (**Fig. 6**). The goal of this joint is to prevent an excessive hyperextension moment during stance, preventing further damage to the joint and posterior joint capsule without buckling. The orthotist can leave a small amount of hyperextension at the joint, so the patient feels secure enough to transfer weight in stance with a smooth transition into swing phase. If the posterior offset is not adequate, a locking knee joint can be used; however, this forces the patient to use a high-energy-consuming compensatory mechanism to advance the limb through swing phase, such as circumduction and/or hip hike.[5]

Drop, or ring, lock

The drop lock is a strong lock and is used in patients with quadriceps weakness (**Fig. 7**). With the leg fully extended, the ring drops down to prevent knee flexion. The knee must be unlocked manually by pulling up to disengage it. The sit-to-stand transition can be challenging for patients with balance impairment.[5]

Bail, or lever, locks

The bail, or lever, lock allows unlocking or locking of the medial and lateral knee joints simultaneously by providing an upward force on the bail, disengaging both locks at the same time (**Fig. 8**). Although this is convenient, it requires that the patient be able to weight shift to the contralateral side without loss of balance, and then, if bumped, the bail may accidently unlock. Addition of a cable to the bail system can prevent accidental unlocking of the knee.[5]

Stance-control knee joints

Stance-control knee joints provide stability during stance phase by preventing the knee from buckling but allow a transition to free swing during swing phase. Stance-control knees are more energy efficient for the polio population because the patients do not have to resort to an energetically costly compensatory mechanism such as circumduction or hip hiking, as with a locked-knee KAFO. The joints can be mechanical

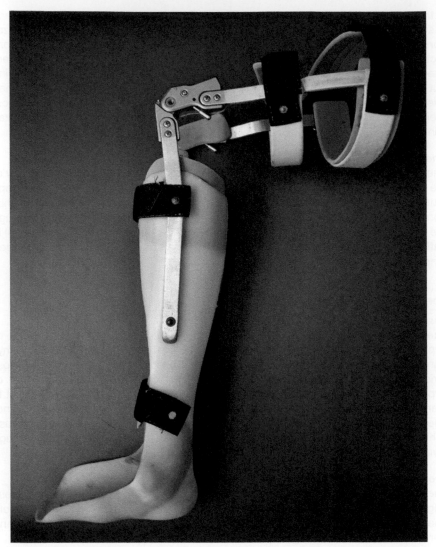

Fig. 6. Custom hybrid KAFO with posterior offset knee hinge, plastic AFO portion, and standard metal thigh section.

or electronic and are likely to require the polio survivors to seek additional gait training after delivery.[5]

Proximal Thigh Section

Standard thigh
A standard thigh section is appropriate for patients with polio with limited ambulation or wearing bilateral bracing (see **Fig. 6**). The limb loading is limited and, if the gait is not adjusted, a standard thigh section is adequate.[5]

Quadrilateral and ischial containment
The use of a quadrilateral or ischial containment design for the proximal thigh section of the KAFO allows the patients with polio to transfer their weight through the

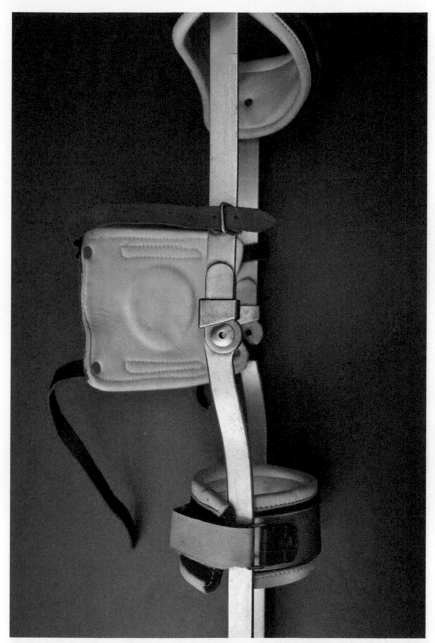

Fig. 7. Custom metal and leather KAFO with drop, or ring, lock.

KAFO during stance phase of gait by unloading the contralateral extremity, putting more weight through the weaker side, and reducing energy expenditure (see **Fig. 8**).[5] The ischial weight-bearing socket design can also provide support to a weak hip.[4]

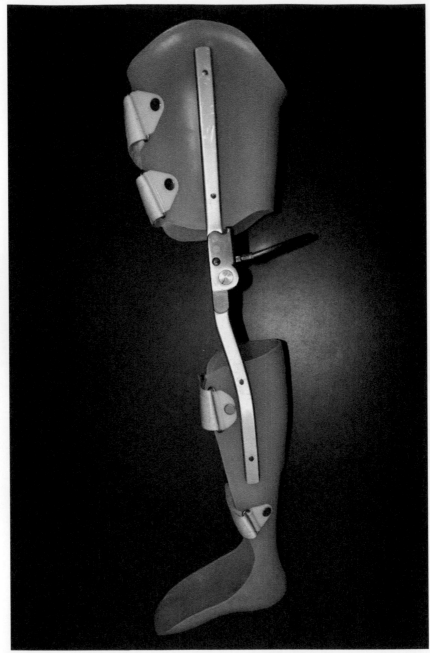

Fig. 8. Custom molded plastic with KAFO bail, or lever, locks and quadrilateral thigh section.

Other Components

Molded inner boot

The molded inner boot design is often used in the pediatric polio population but is beneficial for any patient with severe deformity of the foot and ankle. The molded inner boot allows total contact with a soft plastic material within a rigid AFO section that maintains control while creating pressure relief.[5]

Metal and leather ankle-foot orthoses and knee-ankle-foot orthoses

Traditionally, AFOs and KAFOs for patients with polio were fabricated of metal and leather (**Figs. 9–11**). After years of wear, they mold well to the patients' bodies, making them extremely comfortable and durable. However, metal and leather do not provide the best control of the anatomy during the gait cycle. Patients with polio accustomed to this design may be reluctant to trial a newer design with modern materials, such as thermoplastics and carbon fiber, which can be molded to and better control the soft tissues during gait.[5] Many polio survivors become accustomed to the weight of their devices and they feel supported.[4]

Material choice

Advances in materials science have allowed cost-efficiency and lighter-weight designs. Thermoplastics, carbon fiber, aluminum, and titanium have benefited polio survivors because these materials provide strength while keeping the device as light as possible.[5] It is sometimes difficult convincing a patient to accept a modern plastic brace that is thinner and lighter, but equally supportive.[4]

Bracing for the Upper Extremity in Polio and Postpolio

Dr C.E. Irwin[8] published an article in the *Orthopedic & Prosthetic Appliance Journal* in September 1956 titled "Poliomyelitis: Splints for the Upper Extremity." He states that the splints presented are designed and used for therapeutic reasons only. He notes that he has observed patients with polio with upper extremity involvement develop ingenious substitution patterns and discard equipment. His goal, as an orthopedic surgeon, was to evaluate these patients and perform operative procedures to make them as independent as possible without the need of an apparatus. He recommended that splints for the upper extremity preferably be dynamic, providing support and function simultaneously. Splints for the upper extremity were used in the acute phase, both preoperatively and postoperatively to aid function. The devices he presents include splints for intrinsic hand weakness, weak index finger, weak finger extensors, weak finger flexors, contracture of long finger flexors, wrist drop, stand feeders, and overhead slings.[8]

Shoulder

Shoulder splinting in poliomyelitis was thought to be a controversial subject. The 3 possibly weakened muscle groups are the shoulder abductors, the rotator cuff, and the shoulder depressors.[8]

Elbow

Therapeutically, assistive devices that allowed patients with polio to get the hand to the face by assisting elbow flexion provided patients with the ability to self-feed, brush their teeth, and comb their hair. The apparatus flexed the elbow by a series of overhead slings attached to a wheelchair that were activated by shoulder depression or shifting of body weight toward the hemiparetic side.[8] A variety of neoprene sleeves, with or without stays, can be used for elbow support in the chronic paralysis phase.[4]

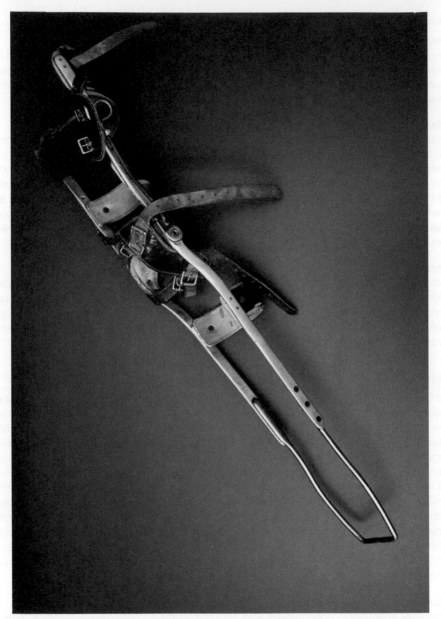

Fig. 9. Custom metal and leather KAFO with round calipers to allow for attachment to multiple shoes. Custom-adapted spring-loaded drop lock for easy unlocking of the knee.

Wrist

Wrist splinting with an off-the shelf wrist-hand orthosis can help protect and position the wrist joint for functional use of the hand.[4] A cock-up splint benefits patients with polio with wrist drop and finger flexor weakness by making use of tenodesis.[8]

Fingers

Splinting of the fingers served to stretch tight muscles to prevent or reduce contractures. Dynamic finger splinting was used to pull or transfer function to a stronger

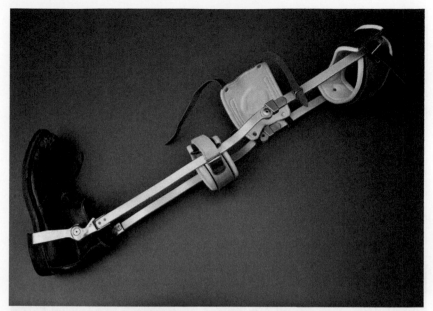

Fig. 10. Metal and leather KAFO with drop lock and stirrup attached to boot (side view).

muscle, such as the first dorsal interosseus.[8] A neoprene or elastic thumb spica splint stabilizes the thumb, reduces pain, and assists with functional pinch.[4]

Risk of Falls/Injury

Polio survivors have symptoms that are known risk factors for falls in the elderly. A study of polio survivors in the Netherlands found that 74% of responders reported at least 1 fall in the past year and 60% reported 2 or more. One-third of patients who had fallen had reduced the amount they walked because of fear of falling. Most reported falls happened (1) in a familiar environment (86%), (2) during ambulation (72%), and (3) in the afternoon (50%). Factors independently associated with both falls and recurrent falls were (1) quadriceps muscle strength of weakest leg (Medical Research Council ≤3), (2) fear of falling, and (3) complaints of problems maintaining balance.[9]

Orthosis Compliance

Compliance with a properly fitted orthosis may reduce falls and prevent injury in polio survivors. Polio-specific considerations that affect compliance are energy conservation, weight of device, body mechanics, and anatomic considerations. Case studies show patients with polio prefer lighter-weight devices and new technologies that offer improved joints and stronger, more customizable braces. In a cross-sectional survey of polio survivors using a custom-made dorsiflexion-restricting AFO of calf muscle weakness, they found that almost three-quarters of the polio survivors were using their orthoses. Fit and comfort affect usability.[10] It is recommended that, in addition to discussing the patient's goals and anticipated improvements with bracing, there should also be a discussion of the orthosis also being a possible hindrance in daily life, because this will help manage expectations and reduce noncompliance.

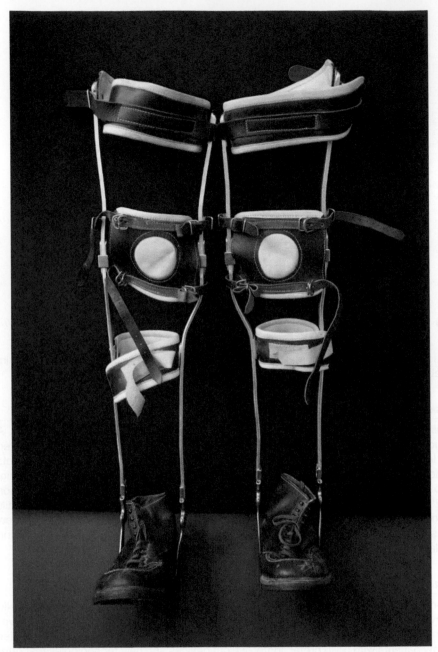

Fig. 11. Bilateral metal and leather KAFOs with drop locks and stirrup attached to boots.

Best Practices

- Assess fall risk with Timed Up and Go (TUG) and Berg Balance Test:
  - The TUG has been studied in community-dwelling elderly people with a variety of medical comorbidities (hypertension, arthritis, low back pain, cancer, heart

Table 1
Cutoff scores indicating risk of falls by population

Population	Cutoff Score: Time(s)	Reference
Community-dwelling adults	>13.5	Shumway-Cook et al,[12] 2000
Older adults already attending a falls clinic	>15	Whitney et al,[13] 2005
Hip osteoarthritis	>10	Arnold et al,[14] 2007

Photos: (custom AFOs and KAFOs device credit Joshua James, BOCPO of South County Artificial Limb & Brace, photographs by Dr. Claudia Wheeler).

Data from Shumway-Cook A, Brauer S, et al. Predicting the probability for falls in community-dwelling older adults using the timed up & go test. Phys Ther 2000; 80(9):896–903, Whitney JC, Lord SR, et al. Streamlining assessment and intervention in a falls clinic using the timed up and go test and physiological profile assessments. Age Ageing 2005;3496:567–71, Arnold CM, Faulkner RA. The history of falls and the association of the timed up and go test to falls and near-falls in older adults with hip osteoarthritis. BMC Geriatr 2007;7:17.

disease, thyroid disease, and diabetes) but not specifically in the postpolio population.

- ○ Steffen and colleagues[11] reported the TUG normative data for community-dwelling adults based on age. For those aged 60 to 69 years, the TUG was 8 seconds; age 70 to 79 years, the TUG was 9 seconds; and 80 to 89 years, the TUG was 10 to 11 seconds. The TUG in this population had excellent test-retest reliability.
- ○ Polio survivors who have TUGs that are greater than a typical community-dwelling elder of similar age may benefit from a dedicated course of therapy to mitigate fall risk.
- It may be useful to reassess the TUG once properly braced and after a course of skilled physical therapy to assess improvement and reduction in fall risk **(Table 1)**.
- The best orthotic results are often achieved with patients who have significant deficits but walk regularly, are well motivated, and are willing and able to adapt their gait for orthotic use.
- Lighter-weight devices provide opportunity for energy conservation.
- Periodic tune-up of a device may be preferable to a new device in patients with polio.

CLINICS CARE POINTS

- Painful ankles in postpolio patients wearing PLS AFOs: if bracing evaluation reveals symptoms consistent with ankle arthritis or painful/decreased ankle ROM, consider a discussion about changing to a solid ankle AFO and rocker bottom sole shoe modification.

- Postpolio patients with leg length discrepancy that is not addressed: the leg length discrepancy may be source of back pain because of secondary scoliosis; consider an evaluation for heel lift, because significant leg length discrepancies may require a lift inside the shoe and additional lift added to the sole.

- Knee hyperextension in patients with postpolio syndrome wearing AFOs: have a discussion addressing the pros and cons of modifications to the current AFO to reduce knee hyperextension versus changing to a KAFO with offset knee joint. A KAFO is more stable but heavier, especially for patients with postpolio syndrome.

DISCLOSURE

The author has nothing to disclose.

REFERENCES

1. Joseph B, Watts H. Polio revisited: reviving knowledge and skills to meet the challenge of resurgence. J Children's Orthopaedics 2015;9(5):325–38.
2. Fowler PT, Botte MJ, Mathewson JW, et al. Energy cost of ambulation with different methods of foot and ankle immobilization. J Orthop Res 1993;11(3):416–21.
3. Hachisuka K, Makino K, Wada F, et al. Oxygen consumption, oxygen cost and physiological cost index in polio survivors: a comparison of walking without orthosis, with an ordinary or carbon-fibre reinforced plastic knee-ankle-foot orthosis. J Rehabil Med 2007;39(8):646–50.
4. Siegel IM. The utility of post-polio bracing. Post-polio Health International. Available at: https://www.polioplace.org/living-with-polio/utility-post-polio-bracing.
5. Lovegreen W, Kwasniewski M, Panchang P, et al. Orthotic management of polio and Postpolio syndrome. In: Chapter 27 in Atlas of Orthoses and Assistive Devices. 5th Edition; 2019.
6. McNalley TE, Yorkston KM, Jensen MP, et al. A review of secondary health conditions in post-polio syndrome: prevalence and effects of aging. Am J Phys Med Rehabil 2015;94(2):139–45.
7. Ploeger HE, Sicco AB, Merel-Anne B, et al. Ankle-foot orthoses that restrict dorsiflexion improve walking in polio survivors with calf muscle weakness. Gait Posture 2014;40(3):391–8.
8. Irwin CE. Poliomyelitis: splints for the upper extremity. Orthop Prosthetic Appliance J 1956;51–60.
9. Bickerstaffe A, Beelen A, Nollet F. Circumstances and consequences of falls in polio survivors. J Rehabil Med 2010;42:908–15.
10. Ploeger HE, Bus SA, Breham MA, et al. Use and usability of custom-made dorsiflexion-restricting ankle foot orthoses for calf muscle weakness in polio survivors: a cross-sectional study. Eur J Phys Med Rehabil 2020;56(5):575–84.
11. Steffen TM, Hacker TA, Mollinger L, et al. Age- and gender-related test performance in community-dwelling elderly people: six-minute walk test , berg balance scale, timed up & go test, and gait speeds. Phys Ther 2002;82(2):128–37.
12. Shumway-Cook A, Brauer S, Woollacott M, et al. Predicting the probability for falls in community-dwelling older adults using the timed up & go test. Phys Ther 2000;80(9):896–903.
13. Whitney JC, Lord SR, Close JCT, et al. Streamlining assessment and intervention in a falls clinic using the timed up and go test and physiological profile assessments. Age Ageing 2005;34(6):567–71.
14. Arnold CM, Faulkner RA. The history of falls and the association of the timed up and go test to falls and near-falls in older adults with hip osteoarthritis. BMC Geriatr 2007;7:17.

Nerve Conduction Study/ Electromyography: Common Neuropathies and Considerations for Patients with Polio

Andrew Dubin, MD, MS

KEYWORDS

- Polio • Postpolio syndrome • Neuromuscular fatigue • Anterior horn cell

KEY POINTS

- Acute poliomyelitis: the pathophysiology of the disease can best be described as more than meets the eye. Typically, the physical examination is consistent with scatter-shot or spotty involvement of the muscle system.
- Postacute polio infection, motor neuron pool makeup: postacute infection with polio resulted in subdivisions of motor recovery.
- Postpolio syndrome (PPS) is multifactorial in cause and potentially includes multiple factors, normal aging and loss of motor units, premature dropout of muscle fibers and motor units (group 3 and 4 motor units), impaired neuromuscular junction function, impaired ability to perform oxidative phosphorylation, with decreased ability to tolerate oxidative stress.
- Common complaints in PPS: fatigue. In approximately 40% of patients with PPS, the fatigue is of a degree that it affects their ability to work or complete work. More than 25% of patients note that the fatigue affects and impairs their ability to perform activities of daily living.

ELECTROMYOGRAPHIC, RESPIRATORY, AND MUSCULOSKELETAL CONSIDERATIONS
History: Why it Is Important to Understand the Illness and its Acute Findings

Acute poliomyelitis is now extremely rare in the United States. Routine vaccination is no longer done because the documented cases in the United States were invariably related to the polio vaccine as opposed to the acute viral infection.

Worldwide there are still sporadic outbreaks, which are typically treated with acute inoculation programs.

The pathophysiology of the disease can best be described as more than meets the eye. Typically, the physical examination is consistent with scatter-shot or spotty involvement of the muscle system. However, the apparent isolation to the muscle

Division of PM&R, Department of Orthopedics and Rehabilitation Medicine, University of Florida, 3450 Hull Road Suite 3301, POB 112727, Gainesville, FL 32611, USA
E-mail address: andrew.dubin@ufl.edu

Phys Med Rehabil Clin N Am 32 (2021) 527–535
https://doi.org/10.1016/j.pmr.2021.02.005
1047-9651/21/© 2021 Elsevier Inc. All rights reserved.

system is in contradistinction to the work by Bodain from the 1940s through 1980s, which described the generalized nature of the disease, despite the clinical presentation of an apparent spotty involvement of the motor system.[1] This dichotomy would be consistent with the observation of subdivided motor unit recovery after acute infection, as well as electromyography (EMG) data and observation that apparently normal neurons might have larger motor unit territories and be subject to slightly shorter life expectancies (group 2 and clearly group 3 motor neurons).[2]

As a classic anterior horn cell disorder, the general theme of painless weakness would be the default thought paradigm when discussing acute poliomyelitis, but one of the most common manifestations of the acute disease was significant muscle tenderness. The additional common findings of positive Babinski and increased deep tendon reflexes raised the question of central nervous system (CNS) involvement.[2,3]

Postacute infection with polio resulted in 5 subdivisions of motor recovery:

1. Normal unaffected neurons away from the area of lost neurons
2. Normal neurons near the area of lost neurons
3. Neurons initially affected but with apparent full recovery
4. Moderately affected neurons that survive but with decreased size
5. Severely affected neurons that fail to fully recover

Morphologically groups 1 and 2 are normal neurons but have larger motor units. Typically their life span is normal to mildly decreased.

Group 3 motor neurons represent a threshold group of motor neurons. Although they appear to have recovered, they are less tolerant of physiologic stress and typically have shorter lifespans than normal motor units.

Group 4 motor neurons clearly have diminished capacity to tolerate physiologic stress and maintain functional synapses, and clearly have decreased life expectancy.

Group 5 motor neurons never exhibit normal function, and, for the duration of their demonstrably shorter life cycle, show abnormal function with significantly impaired tolerance to physiologic stress.[2]

Typical of surviving neurons in postpolio patients, the terminal axons have up to 5 times the number of muscle fibers per motor unit. This finding suggests that recovery of function depends on the degree of terminal arborization and sprouting that leads to the functional recovery, but also helps to shed light on why postpolio develops. This question includes why it might not manifest for decades, and also helps to explain the phenomenon of sudden decline in function in patients who are polio survivors.[2–5]

The magnitude of postpolio syndrome (PPS) is large. It is estimated that, in the United States, there are approximately 1.6 million polio survivors, with about 640,000 of that group having paralytic polio. These data were derived from a 1987 National Health Interview Survey that had specific questions for persons who had been given the diagnosis of polio with or without paralysis.

A position statement from the Postpolio Task Force noted that retrospective studies using objective criteria estimate that PPS develops in 20% to 40% of acute paralytic polio survivors.[2] Extrapolation from these data implies that approximately 200,000 to 400,000 persons are likely to experience signs and symptoms of PPS.[2]

ELECTROMYOGRAPHY FINDINGS, CONSIDERATIONS, AND PITFALLS

Patients with PPS manifest with predictable findings on electrodiagnostic testing. These findings include large amplitude and increased duration of motor units in all involved muscles; however, what is unappreciated is that these findings are also observed in clinically uninvolved muscles, which speaks to the findings of the diffuse nature of the disease, even though the clinical and physical examination findings seem to be more scattered.[2,3,6]

With regard to more nuanced EMG, single-fiber needle EMG shows increased jitter and blocking in both stable muscles as well as newly weakened muscles. The histologic correlates for abnormal jitter is the expression of N-CAM (neural cell adhesion molecule), which is expressed in muscle fibers that have acutely lost innervation. Muscle fibers that fail to achieve functional reinnervation lose the expression of N-CAM and eventually atrophy.[2,7]

Clearly these findings fail to fully explain the nearly ubiquitous and early findings of fatigue in the muscles of patients with PPS. Although the exact mechanism or mechanisms at play have not yet been fully elucidated, it seems that a myriad of factors coalesce to create the phenomenology associated with PPS.

Possible factors include normal aging and loss of motor units, premature dropout of muscle fibers and motor units (group 3 and 4 motor units, possibly even group 1 and 2), impaired neuromuscular junction function, impaired oxidative phosphorylation with decreased ability to tolerate oxidative stress, and (at the speculative end of the theoretic continuum) potential immune dysregulation with active ongoing damage to motor neurons, and possible persistent polio virus RNA and potential mutants causing persistent smoldering infection.[2,5,8]

Aging is a normal process and the loss of motor neurons with normal aging is well established. Typically this does not occur until after age 60 years, although postpolio motor neurons may have a shortened life span, and in many cases is closely related to the degree of abnormality of the survival pool of recovered neurons. As such, risk factors for early dropout include earlier age of injury and heavier metabolic loads. Immune-mediated phenomenon or immune dysregulation has also been proposed as a mechanism based on autopsy data obtained from patients known to have had polio but who died years later from non–polio-related events. Findings of inflammation of the perivascular area of gray matter in the spinal cord and gliosis disproportionate to the degree of neuronal loss correlate with a potential ongoing immune-mediated inflammatory process. Muscle biopsy data revealing cluster of differentiation (CD) 4+ and CD8+ cells around healthy muscle fibers with major histocompatibility complex 1 (MHC-1) expression further raises the specter of inflammation, because this pattern of findings can also be seen in some inflammatory myopathies. In addition, the expression of MHC-1 is similar to the expression seen in acute polio infection, and the presence of immunoglobulin-M antiganglioside antibody in patients with PPS is also seen in acute polio infection. All of these findings potentially implicate a dysregulation of the immune system and also hint at a possible low-level inflammatory process.[2,5,8]

The theory and argument suggesting the possible role for persistent poliovirus are more speculative and face many challenges. The most significant factors countering this potential option include the well-documented monophasic nature of the disease without a clear reactivation syndrome and the highly lytic nature of the virus in culture. This constellation of findings make persistent infection highly unlikely. The alternative is that there are models of persistent infection in animals and in immune-compromised human hosts, and that, theoretically, a model could be created of a dormant, possibly mutant, version of the RNA that activates years later in the CNS and results in the low-grade immune response previously described. Although theoretically possible, this is highly speculative and, to date, there are no conclusive data to suggest this.[2,5,7,8]

The findings noted in PPS indicate that the deterioration is an active and ongoing process involving the spinal motor neurons, resulting in ongoing denervation and continual remodeling of terminal axons. Ultimately the balance between denervation and reinnervation inexorably tips toward denervation becoming dominant, with the predictable sequelae of atrophy and progressive weakness.

Fatigue is noted in more than 90% of patients with PPS (as discussed elsewhere in this issue). In approximately 40% of patients with PPS, the fatigue affects their ability to work or complete work. More than 25% of patients note that the fatigue affects and impairs their ability to perform activities of daily living (ADLs).

Although the clinical manifestations of acute polio infection seem to be predominately peripheral, in most cases there is also significant CNS involvement. Damage to the thalamus, hypothalamus, putamen, globus pallidus, caudate, cerebellum, substantia nigra, and components of the reticular activating system is well documented and typical.[2–4,9]

The findings of lethargy, somnolence, and even coma during the acute infection correlate with severe involvement of the reticular formation, locus ceruleus, thalamus, and hypothalamus. It has been hypothesized that progression of damage in these areas, along with aging, explain the central fatigue noted by patients with PPS. The age-related loss of neurons in these regions may reach a critical threshold and result in impaired reticular formation activation, which may explain the fatigue and mild cognitive impairment shown in patients with PPS. The use of dopaminergic agents may have utility in PPS for central fatigue. Its efficacy has been shown in patients with chronic fatigue syndrome and there are data to suggest an overlap in the pathology of the two syndromes.[2]

DIAGNOSIS OF POSTPOLIO SYNDROME AND RELATION TO ELECTROMYOGRAPHY

The diagnosis of PPS can present challenges. As previously discussed, there are no specific confirmatory tests. Therefore, the history and physical examination are of paramount importance. Confirming the original diagnosis of poliomyelitis is critical. The extent, namely the muscle groups involved, and the severity of the deficits during the acute infection and then the extent of recovery are all critical elements.

Once the extent, severity, and recovery data have been obtained, the next step in the history gathering should focus on establishing a timeline of the patient's functional capacity over time, and whether deficits that are now manifesting are gradual in onset, abrupt, or intermittent.

In all cases, it is important to delve into the history in an attempt to rule out mimics and masqueraders, such as focal compression neuropathy, myopathies, diffuse toxic-metabolic neuropathy (diabetic, drug induced, chemotherapy, and so forth), neuromuscular junction defects, or superimposed CNS (brain and/or spinal cord) processes such as cerebrovascular accident, diffuse small vessel disease, CNS demyelinating disorders, or spondylotic radiculomyelopathy.

The hallmark complaint of new-onset weakness in patients with PPS can be seen in previously weak muscles as well as clinically unaffected muscles. Respiratory and bulbar muscles can be affected, and questions regarding pulmonary function, swallowing, and chewing should be included in the history and data gathering.

An interesting observation in patients with PPS is that greater than one-third note new-onset cold intolerance.[2–4]

As with any nerve conduction study/EMG evaluation, the physical examination is focused on a detailed neuromusculoskeletal examination. The goal is to assess the distribution and severity of involvement. Careful examination of previously clinically unaffected muscles should be undertaken, because they may now start to reveal the extent of damage incurred during the acute phase of polio many years prior. They may now manifest with subtle weakness or even more commonly impaired tolerance for repetitive activity.[2–4]

Careful observation of the patient is needed, and so all patients examined for potential PPS should be examined in a gown. Atrophy and fasciculations, when present, should be noted and their distribution recorded in detail. Deep tendon reflexes should be suppressed to absent and sensation should be preserved, although profoundly weak atrophic limbs may show paradoxic increased sensation.

Sudden appearance of hyperreflexia in a weak, atrophic limb should raise the question of a potential CNS process as the potential driver of new weakness and warrants further investigation with appropriate imaging studies.

Laboratory data tend to be normal except for possible subtle increase in creatine kinase level, particularly after exercise. Significant increase should stimulate investigation for underlying myopathy. To evaluate for possible masqueraders and mimics, complete blood count to evaluate for anemia, thyroid studies to assess for possible thyroid dysfunction, and rheumatologic studies to evaluate for possible immune/inflammatory disorders are reasonable.

Imaging studies, including computed tomography/MRI of the brain and spinal cord, to assess for primary brain disorders and spinal cord–level abnormalities, including compressive myelopathy or root level impingement, are appropriate. Electrodiagnostic evaluation (EDX) studies to evaluate for focal compression neuropathy or radiculopathy are also appropriate, as well as EDX testing to evaluate for possible polyneuropathy. In essence, laboratory imaging and EDX data are used to rule out other possible explanations for the complaints that patients with PPS are noting. The diagnosis of PPS is a diagnosis of exclusion.[2–4]

RESPIRATORY FINDINGS AND CONSIDERATIONS

Pulmonary dysfunction in patients with PPS presents many challenges. Impaired pulmonary function can be a direct consequence of the pathophysiology underlying PPS, but of equal if not greater importance is the interplay between PPS and common disorders such a chronic obstructive pulmonary disease, asthma, and congestive heart failure.[2,9–11] The recent introduction of coronavirus disease 2019 (COVID-19) and the phenomenon of paucisymptomatic COVID infection introduces another layer of complexity to managing postpolio patients with pulmonary dysfunction.

The evaluation of a patient with known polio as a child who presents decades later with pulmonary dysfunction requires in-depth evaluation to determine whether there are elements of reactive airway disease, emphysema, or chronic bronchitis contributing to the issue, or whether these are the major stand-alone issues. Ventilatory muscle fatigue can manifest with decreased lung volumes, compromise in maximal inspiratory and expiratory pressures, and decreased peak airflow and cough flow rates. Impaired pulmonary muscle function results in chronic hypoventilation, decreased lung volumes, low-level chronic atelectasis, decreased lung compliance, and increased chest wall stiffness. Exacerbating factors can include extrinsic issues such as scoliosis (which further affects lung volumes), atelectasis, and decreased chest wall compliance.

Impaired cough flow increases risk for compromised pulmonary secretion management, and a decrease in inspiratory capacity to less than 2.5 L increases risk for failure to adequately clear airway secretions. This condition increases risk for respiratory compromise. A major parameter to ensure safe management of airway secretions is peak cough flow. Values more than 3 L/s are needed to maintain safe airway secretion management. When values decrease below that threshold, assisted cough techniques, both manual and mechanical, should be considered.

The goal for patients with PPS is to optimize pulmonary function, through early identification and intervention, and to avoid hospitalization, intubation, and need for mechanical ventilation. The timely use of noninvasive ventilatory assist strategies and education in self-monitoring can all help maintain quality of life. Interventions such as glossopharyngeal breathing can be lifesaving, because it is effective, patient controlled, and fully portable. The downside is the need for patient training, and it is only useful when the patient is awake. Intermittent positive pressure ventilation is another option for assisted ventilatory support. It is reliable, well tolerated, and noninvasive. However, it is noisy, expensive, and noncosmetic.[2,9–11]

Negative pressure ventilation, or cuirass ventilation, is physiologic, reliable, and helps maintain chest wall compliance. However, it has drawbacks, because it can only be used effectively when supine, and it is less tolerated. If invasive management is required with tracheostomy and ventilator, benefits include high degree of reliability and airway access for secretion management. However, major negatives include invasiveness, tolerability, loss of speech without use of Passy Muir Valve, secondary sequelae such as tracheomalacia and tracheal perforation, and potential increase of pulmonary infection.

Consultation with pulmonary medicine can be helpful in the management and optimization of pulmonary function and tolerance for pulmonary rehabilitation. Cardiology input regarding myocardial performance is critical as well, because heart failure, either with reduced or preserved ejection fraction, can all compromise pulmonary function in PPS. Millions of adults in the United States have heart failure, increasing as time progresses, comparing 2009 to 2012 data with 2013 to 2016 data. This finding includes information sourced from the American Heart Association in conjunction with the National Institutes of Health, implicating increasing prevalence with aging of the population.[2–4,9–12]

Because polio's primary manifestations are muscular during the acute phase of the illness, and subsequent musculoskeletal issues develop secondary to muscle imbalances and disproportionate growth of affected limbs, it is not surprising that, with normal physiologic aging, there may be musculoskeletal complaints. These issues inevitably manifest in patients with PPS. Despite the use of braces for protection, alignment, and support, and despite the use of lifts to correct limb length discrepancies, one of the most common complaints noted by patients with PPS is pain in the muscles, bones, and joints surrounding the muscles that were affected by polio. Approximately one-third to three-quarters of patients with PPS note musculoskeletal pain and about one-quarter note the pain to be severe enough as to negatively affect their ability to perform ADLs and general daily activity levels.[2–4]

Critical evaluation of the patient is needed to assess potential causes of worsening pain. Overuse of affected musculature is a common cause, and education in energy conservation, use of adaptive equipment, and evaluation for new bracing can all have a positive impact on the patient's quality of life.

Education on the use of the Borg Rating Scale of Perceived Exertion for patients with PPS can be helpful. Using the scale with the goal of ending an activity when it increases to a 14 on the scale allows patients to pace their activity and take rest breaks at more appropriate time intervals. It can be challenging to get patients with PPS to accept new bracing or a change in their old bracing to more lightweight and energy-efficient bracing, but education and robust discussion can result in satisfying outcomes over the long term (as discussed elsewhere in this issue). From a practical standpoint, open-ended questions can be effective in starting the conversation. Asking what the patient has noted over the past 2 to 5 years can give insight into areas of particular concern. Questions regarding new-onset or worsening weakness, fatigue, or difficulty in performing ADLs; new or worsening pain; and the impact on quality of life help to quickly establish a patient specific prioritized list. This approach also establishes and builds an effective patient-physician relationship[2] (**Table 1**).

In some instances, total joint replacement for profoundly affected joints can be considered, but special attention needs to be placed on detailed evaluation of the musculature crossing the joint and ultimately controlling the joint.[2] The need for more constrained joint replacement options may need to be considered in evaluating the balance between pain relief and function.

Osteoporosis and associated fracture risk increase as a normal function of aging, and the PPS population is at increased risk because underlying neurologic conditions that result in limb weakness only serve to accelerate the process. Causes for the increased fracture risk include disuse atrophy. In adults who had polio as a child, failure to achieve peak bone mass in the affected limbs and abnormal development of the affected limbs contribute to increased risk. There is no associated increase in the risk for fracture with the use of assistive devices or bracing (Mayo Clinic data). Typical interventions to mitigate fracture risk are appropriate for the PPS population. These strategies include home assessment and evaluation as part of a fall mitigation strategy, calcium supplementation, vitamin D supplementation if needed, hormone replacement therapy as warranted, and gentle progressive weight-bearing exercises.[2]

Treatment of patients with PPS can be challenging. Reports of positive impact on issues of muscle weakness, central fatigue, and decline in cognitive function have been published in the literature with the use of agents that improve neuromuscular

Table 1		
Patients with postpolio syndrome		
Questions	**Complaints**	**Potential Interventions**
What changes have you noted over the past several years?	Increased fatigue	Energy conservation: use of Borg Scale of Perceived Exertion
Are you noting increased fatigue?	Increased pain	Pulmonary and cardiology evaluations to identify potential treatable underlying disorders affecting activity tolerance
Are you having more pain?	Decreased ambulation tolerance: fatigue	
Has your quality of life/ enjoyment changed? If so, in what ways?	Orthopedic	
Are you more sedentary/ less active? If so, why?		Consideration for CNS active agents: dopaminergic agents
		Discussion regarding bracing and consideration for new options when appropriate
		Consideration for possible joint replacement in selected patients
		Appropriate bracing or modification of current bracing system if applicable

junction transmission, increase CNS levels of dopamine (see **Table 1**), and increase insulin growth factor 1 levels. To date, no large, randomized, placebo-controlled studies have shown that any of these interventional strategies have a positive impact on the PPS. There has been some suggestion that dopaminergic agents may be helpful for central fatigue, and larger studies are clearly needed. Prednisone in high doses has also been investigated, with similar nonefficacy noted, and clearly the long-term consequences of high-dose prednisone are such that it would not be a viable option even if some degree of efficacy were noted.

Exercise can be very helpful in the management of pain and muscle weakness. In general, low-intensity exercise programs using lower and or upper extremity ergometry are well tolerated. Aquatic exercise and swimming have a long track record of efficacy and should be encouraged. More controversial is the use of high-intensity exercise. Data from Einarsson[13] reveal that, in a group of patients with PPS who underwent a 12-week high-intensity program of quadriceps strengthening using isokinetic and isometric modes of exercise, significant improvements in strength were noted. This finding suggests that high-intensity exercise can be beneficial when coupled with adequate rest and recovery periods.[2,9]

Poliomyelitis as a disease has been conquered. However, its late-onset manifestations remain a challenge and will remain a challenge for years to come. Physiatrists are uniquely positioned to have a positive impact on this group of patients, both in treating the patients as well as coordinating care from other specialists to optimize functional outcomes and quality of life.

CLINICS CARE POINTS

- Diagnosis of PPS: there are no specific confirmatory tests. The history and physical examination are of paramount importance. Confirming the original diagnosis of poliomyelitis is critical. The muscle groups involved and extent of involvement, during the acute infection and then the extent of recovery, are all critical elements.

- Pulmonary dysfunction in PPS: ventilatory muscle fatigue can manifest with decreased lung volumes, compromise in maximal inspiratory and expiratory pressures, and decreased peak airflow and cough flow rates. Exacerbating factors can include extrinsic issues such as scoliosis, which further affects lung volumes; atelectasis; and chest wall compliance.

- Osteoporosis and associated fracture risk are increased in the PPS population because underlying neurologic conditions that result in limb weakness only serve to accelerate the process. Causes for the increased fracture risk include disuse atrophy and, in adults who had polio as a child, failure to achieve peak bone mass in the affected limbs as well as abnormal development of the affected limbs. Typical interventions to mitigate fracture risk in the general aging population are appropriate for the PPS population. These strategies include home assessment and evaluation as part of a fall mitigation strategy; calcium and vitamin D supplementation; hormone replacement therapy, if needed and appropriate: and gentle progressive weight-bearing exercises as tolerated.

- Acute flaccid myelitis (AFM): AFM is a rare disorder that most commonly affects children, although it has been reported in adults.

- Diagnosis of AFM: diagnostic criteria include acute onset of focal or multifocal flaccid limb weakness and MRI showing spinal cord lesion/lesions that are largely restricted to gray matter and spanning 1 or more spinal segments, regardless of age. Most cases have been reported in individuals less than 21 years of age. Specific exclusions include gray matter lesions secondary to physician-diagnosed malignancy, vascular malformations, or other clearly identifiable anatomic or structural lesions/abnormalities.

DISCLOSURE

Nothing to disclose.

REFERENCES

1. Bodian D. Histopathologic basis of clinical findings in Poliomyelitis. Am J Med 1949;6:563–78.
2. Matthew NB, Omura A. Aging in Polio. Phys Med Rehabil Clin N Am 2005;16: 197–218.
3. Halstead LS. Diagnosing postpolio syndrome, inclusion and exclusion criteria in Silver JK. In: Gawne AC, editor. Postpolio syndrome. First Edition. Philadelphia: Hanley and Belfus; 2004. p. 1–20.
4. Jubelt B, Agre JC. Characteristics and management of postpolio syndrome. JAMA 2000;284:412–4.
5. Boyer F-C, Rapin A, Laffoont I, et al. Post-polio syndrome: pathophysiological hypotheses, diagnosis criteria, drug therapy. Ann Phys Rehabil Med 2010;53(1): 34–41.
6. Trojan DA, Gendron D, Cashman NR. Electrophysiology and electrodiagnosis of the post-polio motor unit. Orthopedics 1991;14(12):1353–61.
7. Maier A, McGreevy A, Timothy B. Molecular pathogenicity of enteroviruses causing neurological disease. Front Microbiol 2020;11:540.
8. Tiffreau V, Rapin A, Serafi R, et al. Post - polio syndrome and rehabilitation. Ann Phys Rehabil Med 2010;53(1):42–50.
9. Shoseyov D, Cohen-Kaufman T, Schwartz I, et al. Comparison of activity and fatigue of the respiratory muscles and pulmonary characteristics between post-polio patients and controls: a pilot study. PLoS One 2017;12:e0182036.
10. Bach JR, Rajaraman R, Ballanger F, et al. Neuromuscular ventilatory insufficiency: effect of home mechanical ventilator use v oxygen therapy on pneumonia and hospitalization rates. Am J Phys Med Rehabil 1998;77(1):8–19.
11. Putcha N, Bradley Drummond M, Wise RA, et al. Comorbidities and chronic obstructive pulmonary disease: prevalence, influence on outcomes, and management. Semin Respir Crit Care Med 2015;36(4):575–91.
12. Evenson KR, Butler EN, Rosamond WD. Prevalence of physical activity and sedentary behavior among adults with cardiovascular disease. J Cardiopulm Rehabil Prev 2014;34(6):406–19.
13. Einarssen G. Muscle Conditioning in late poliomyelitis. Arch Phys Med Rehabil 1991;72:11–4.

Joint and Back Pain
Medications and Role of Injection Therapy for Destructive Joint

Angela Samaan, DO[a],*, Miguel X. Escalon, MD, MPH[b]

KEYWORDS

• Postpolio syndrome • Pain • Postpolio syndrome treatment

KEY POINTS

- Pain is the most characteristic feature of postpolio syndrome (PPS) and has a significant impact on patients' quality of life.
- Symptoms of pain can often be severe, and thorough history and physical examination with referral to providers with expertise are important when approaching patients with PPS pain.
- First-line therapy includes lifestyle changes, physiotherapy, massage therapy, and a variety of exercise and conditioning programs.
- Medications, such as nonsteroidal anti-inflammatory drugs, anticonvulsants, narcotics, and cannabinoids, have been shown to be efficacious in treating pain in PPS; alternate therapies have been or are being investigated, such as intravenous immunoglobulin and L-citrulline.
- More invasive approaches, such as steroid injections, nerve blocks, and arthroplasty, have been used with success for more refractory cases.

INTRODUCTION/EPIDEMIOLOGY

Poliovirus, a neurotropic enterovirus, is a viral infectious disease that can result in damage of motor neurons of the spinal cord and brainstem. In patients with major viremia, destruction of motor neurons occurs and can cause cell death and paralysis of muscle fibers supplied by the affected motor neuron.[1] Paralytic polio is characterized by severe back, joint, and muscle pain, and the development of motor weakness. However, owing to vaccination, poliovirus no longer poses the worldwide public health threat it once did.[2,3] Nonetheless, small areas in the world continue to report cases of poliomyelitis.[4,5] Furthermore, survivors of poliomyelitis live with static neuromuscular

[a] Department of Rehabilitation and Human Performance, Icahn School of Medicine at Mount Sinai, One Gustave L. Levy Place, Box 1240, New York, NY 10029, USA; [b] Icahn School of Medicine at Mount Sinai, 5 East 98th Street, Sixth Floor, Box 1240B, New York, New York 10029, USA
* Corresponding author.
E-mail address: Angela.samaan@mountsinai.org

Phys Med Rehabil Clin N Am 32 (2021) 537–546
https://doi.org/10.1016/j.pmr.2021.02.006
1047-9651/21/© 2021 Elsevier Inc. All rights reserved.
pmr.theclinics.com

sequelae of polio, or postpolio syndrome (PPS). More than 50% of individuals with a history of acute poliomyelitis experience new health problems later in life. The onset of new symptoms occurs approximately 35 years after the initial polio episode, but the delay can range between 8 and 71 years.[6] PPS is more likely to occur in women, patients with severe symptoms during original infection, patients of older age during original infection, and patients with greater recovery after original infection, possibly because of failure of the compensatory processes that facilitated the initial recovery.[5,6]

PPS is commonly characterized by pain. Muscle pain occurs in 38% to 86% of patients; joint pain occurs in 42% to 80% of patients, and nerve compression syndromes result in pain in 49% of patients. Twenty-five percent of patients with PPS report that pain has a significant impact on their daily lives.[7] Muscle pain can be due to postpolio muscle pain resulting from cramps, spasms, fasciculations, and overuse. Joint pain may be caused by joint and soft tissue abnormalities resulting in biomechanical pain. Chronic weakness as a result of acute infection and PPS can produce overuse of certain joints and muscles, which may subsequently result in pain. If polio occurred in childhood, uneven limb size or failed surgical intervention may contribute to pain owing to long-term musculoskeletal degeneration and skeletal asymmetry.[7,8] Furthermore, research has shown polio survivors with significant lower-extremity weakness commonly present with upper-extremity pain secondary to overuse, particularly shoulder pain when shoulders are stressed beyond their physiologic limits.[9,10] Patients with lower-extremity weakness require additional upper-extremity support to ambulate, often with assistance devices, such as crutches. Use of crutches or assistance devices can lead to strain on the upper extremities and pain. In 1 cross-sectional study, joint pain was significantly associated with the degree of initial motor unit involvement as assessed by a subjective increased weakness during initial polio infection and a greater lower-extremity weakness at study presentation.[11]

In a sample of 150 polio survivors, 80% of those surveyed complained of pain. Most commonly reported was pain from the joints of the extremities, followed by pain from the lower back.[11] In 1 study, the most frequent sites of pain were shoulders, lower back, legs, and hips. Sites with the highest average pain intensity included knees, legs, wrists, lower back, and head. Furthermore, participants reported experiencing pain at an earlier age in the legs and chest compared with other pain sites. With regard to pain intensity, persons with PPS have reported levels of pain severity significantly higher than national norms on the bodily pain subscale of the SF-36. Pain is not only common in persons with PPS but also tends to be rated as moderate to severe, tends to occur in many locations, and leads to disruptions in daily living.[5,11]

WHY WE CARE?

PPS is rarely life threatening; however, addressing and controlling pain in PPS are important when treating patients with PPS.[5] Studies have shown that the symptoms of PPS can make it difficult for an affected person to function independently.[7] In studies on disability in patients with PPS, pain symptoms have been shown to impact mobility-related activities.[12] One study showed that the experience of pain was related to the level of physical activity, with more than 50% of the individuals reporting daily pain that was most evident during physical activity.[11] Pain has been shown to interfere with multiple aspects of daily life, notably sleep and recreational activities. The presence of muscle and joint pain is associated with significant reductions in quality of life.[12–14] Therefore, addressing the symptoms, particularly pain, of patients with late effects of polio is key to managing the disease process.

DIAGNOSIS/EVALUATION

Pain secondary to PPS is a clinical diagnosis.[15] One study found that patients commonly described pain in polio-affected limbs as "cramping" or "aching"; however, other descriptive characteristics were used to describe pain quality.[11,16] Patients with PPS and joint pain are more likely to be younger, have had greater subjective weakness during acute polio infection, have a higher body mass index, have lower isometric muscle strength in the lower extremities, and score lower on a general health scale than those who survived polio but did not develop PPS pain.[6] Common pain sites include shoulders, lower back, legs, and hips.[11] Pain may be accompanied by sleep disturbance, gait disturbance, or "flat back syndrome," which is the inability to stand erect because of forward flexion and pain in the lower back and lower extremities.[8,15] Pain is usually exacerbated by overuse and therefore is more commonly worse at the end of the day. In patients with severe viremia, as previously discussed, sequalae of infection may involve residual limb deformity with associated joint destruction, contractures, or ligamentous laxity.[16,17]

Postpolio pain may present as a symptom of PPS; therefore, it is important to identify criteria of this syndrome, including a prior episode with evidence of residual motor neuron loss, a period of 15 years since the onset of acute polio, gradual onset of new weakness and abnormal muscle fatiguability that persists for 1 year, and exclusion of other medical conditions.[18] Patients may be evaluated using tests, including laboratory studies, imaging, electromyography, and nerve conduction studies or muscle biopsy, to rule out other potential diagnoses. Routine laboratory studies tend to be normal in patients with PPS but may be helpful in excluding some systemic diseases.[16] Muscle ultrasound may be helpful in evaluating disease progression and severity by identifying muscle degeneration.[15] Electromyography is useful by confirming prior poliomyelitis infection and by excluding other neuromuscular conditions. Although not frequently obtained, a muscle biopsy may also be helpful in identifying prior poliomyelitis infection in the setting where diagnosis is in question.[7,16]

TREATMENT

Once polio has been established as the cause of a patient's pain, different treatment options may be pursued. Nonpharmacologic treatments include rehabilitation that includes lifestyle changes, physiotherapy, training programs, and avoidance of secondary complications[19] (Box 1). Notably, avoidance of strenuous and fatiguing activity is encouraged with rehabilitation programs, as such activities may result in decreased muscle strength, fatigue, and pain.[19,20] Weight loss programs can often aid in pain control, as excess weight can burden joints, which will further exacerbate symptoms.[12] Nonetheless, various rehabilitation strategies are possible for treatment of postpolio pain. Balneotherapy is the most tolerated.[20] Muscular strengthening is possible if it is moderate, and tolerance is evaluated regularly. The combination of reducing strenuous activities with carefully prescribed and monitored progressive resistance exercises and cardiopulmonary conditioning has been shown to reverse weakness and reduce fatigue.[19–22] For patients requiring assistive devices for weak or painful joints, it is important to evaluate old braces, canes, or crutches and prescribe appropriate devices that limit fatigue in order to reduce pain symptoms while maintaining function.[22,23] An assessment by a physiatrist or physician specializing in PPS can aid in determining the appropriate changes needed to optimize patient benefits from assistive devices.

When conservative measures, including rest and rehabilitation, fail to improve pain, pharmacologic treatment is indicated[19] (Table 1). A retrospective cross-sectional

---

Box 1
Nonpharmacologic/conservative therapies in treatment of postpolio pain

Nonpharmacologic therapies

Lifestyle changes

Physiotherapy

Physical therapy

Massage therapy

Heat

Ice

Assistive devices

Bracing and brace modifications

Weight loss

Strength training/resistance exercises

Cardiopulmonary conditioning

Biofeedback training

Counseling

---

survey identified several treatments used by patients with postpolio pain and high-lighted which percent of patients was maintained on such therapies and their level of relief. Initial treatment with nonsteroidal anti-inflammatory drugs (NSAIDs) and acet-aminophen was noted in more than 70% of all patients, with an average relief rating of 4.5 on a 10-point pain scale.[11] Patients with severe pain have greater pain relief with these same medications. Alternative pharmacologic therapies are also used when indicated in patients without appropriate relief. Tricyclic antidepressants are often a second-line pharmacotherapy that offers a modest improvement in patients' pain. Such medications, although helpful, have unfavorable side-effect profiles and are not often used for an extended duration. Gabapentin, a medication used for various pain syndromes, offers a more tolerable option for pain management. Its use has been shown to be less effective in reducing pain symptoms than NSAIDs and acet-aminophen and is less commonly prescribed in postpolio pain.[19]

Many medications have shown improvement in joint pain and offer promising results in patient care. Several anticonvulsants have been used in treating pain in polio. Although phenytoin offers only mild improvement in symptoms, carbamazepine and lamotrigine showed more favorable results.[11] When surveyed, patients with moderate pain using carbamazepine identified a significant improvement in symptoms. In addi-tion, lamotrigine has been identified as a well-tolerated medicine with notable symp-toms improvement. Open trials of lamotrigine in patients led to statistically significant improvements in pain, quality of life, and fatigue. Sample sizes in studies of both car-bamazepine and lamotrigine were small; however, they present promising results. Similarly, diazepam also presented positive results in controlling moderate pain, although it is less used owing to side effects and issues with tolerability.[11,12]

Controlled medications have been trialed in postpolio pain. Narcotics are used often in postpolio pain, in both average pain and refractory, severe cases. Narcotics have been shown to have the greatest level of pain relief in patients surveyed in cross-sectional analysis. One study reviewed 25 different therapies and compared pain relief in patients with moderate and severe pain. Narcotics offered the highest pain relief

Table 1
Pharmacologic and interventional therapies in treatment of postpolio pain

Therapy	Pain Control	Notes
NSAIDs/acetaminophen	Moderate	Greater impact in patients with severe symptoms
Tricyclic antidepressants	Mild	Unfavorable side-effect profile
Diazepam	Moderate	Unfavorable side effects; risk of dependence
Gabapentin	Minimal-mild	Well tolerated but less effective
Phenytoin	Mild	Side effects may outweigh benefits
Carbamazepine	Moderate-significant	Limited data on its use
Lamotrigine	Moderate-significant	Limited data on its use
Narcotics	Significant	Unfavorable side effects; risk of dependence; patients must be closely monitored
Marijuana	Moderate-significant	Greater impact in those with severe symptoms
Steroids ± amantadine	Minimal	Side effects outweigh benefits; may have limited benefit for short-term relief
Pyridostigmine	Minimal	Conflicting data on efficacy
Modafinil	None	Compared with placebo
Coenzyme Q10	Minimal	Minimal data supporting use
Intravenous immunoglobulin (IVIg)	Mild-moderate	Multiple studies with conflicting data; overall cost may outweigh benefits
L-citrulline	Moderate	Limited data; currently under investigation
Steroid injections	Mild-moderate	Limited data; used often in refractory patients with refractory symptoms
Nerve blocks	Significant	Limited data
Intrathecal analgesia	Mild-moderate	Only studied in case reports
Static magnetic fields	Moderate	Limited data on its use
Acupuncture	Mild-moderate	Cost-effective with minimal risk
Joint arthroplasty	Significant	High risk; may have benefit in refractory cases. Given risks, refer to orthopedics specialized in PPS

score of all therapies studied. More than half of the patients in the study were placed on narcotics for pain relief. The average patient noted a pain relief score of 8.11 out of 10.[11] Although such results were noted, side-effect profiles make such medications difficult to use long term, with concerns for dependence issues. Nearly one-third of patients who were on narcotics was continued on them chronically.[12,22] Smaller samples of patients have been tried on medicinal marijuana. Although overall number of studied patients was small, marijuana has been shown to be affective in both average and severe cases.[11,19]

Several studies have been performed to find treatment options for refractory pain symptoms.[24] Much of these studies have been aimed at targeting inflammatory changes identified in PPS. Elevated inflammatory markers and cytokines have been noted in joint spaces of patients, which postulate a likely systemic response leading to this syndrome.[7] These observations on the pathogenesis of postpolio pain were used to serve as targets for therapeutic approaches in several trials.[22,24] Treatment for the systemic inflammatory response was initially studied in the 1990s in trials of predni-sone in combination with amantadine to target pain and fatigue. Trials showed the risks of steroids, including weight gain, poor glycemic control, myopathy, and osteo-porosis, outweighed the minimal benefit provided. Short-term steroid use has shown some benefit in improving muscle strength without meaningful functional improve-ment.[11,19,22] Other therapies studied, unfortunately, had little improvement as well. Randomized trials of pyridostigmine have been conflicting and have not proved to be of benefit in improving pain, strength, or quality of life. Similarly, modafinil has shown benefit when compared with placebo, and coenzyme Q10 had a similar lack of positive results.[22]

More recent trials have looked at identifying newer treatment options. Intravenous immunoglobulin (IVIg) has been 1 therapy that has been more widely studied and iden-tified as a promising treatment. IVIg has been used for decades in neurologic autoim-mune disorders, yet its clinical effects have not been completely understood. There are several proposed mechanisms on how IVIg helps in many conditions, most notably its effect on cytokine production when pertaining to inflammatory pain control. Research on neuroimmunomodulation showed that IVIg reduced cerebrospinal fluid in-flammatory cytokine levels in patients with PPS. These findings led to several studies that examined IVIg for pain management in PPS. Two separate randomized trials concluded that patients treated with IVIg had significant improvements in muscle strength and improvements in pain. Furthermore, a third trial showed improvement in overall quality of life in treated patients compared with placebo. These studies are promising; however, limitations are noted as optimal dosing, and therapy cycle is un-known, as each study used different dosing and varying number of treatments. IVIg also comes with a great financial cost, and its widespread use may be limited in light of this. These studies, although presenting positive results, are limited and do not pro-vide sufficient support to its standard use given its cost. Nonetheless, owing to a favor-able side-effect profile, IVIg may offer a unique, therapeutic option for pain in PPS and can be further researched.[25–30] In addition, a single-center, double-blinded randomized controlled trial on L-citrulline is being investigated. It has preliminarily shown benefit in muscular dystrophies in improving endurance and is now being studied in PPS.[22]

There are scant data to support the role of more invasive means of pain control in patients with PPS. The evidence is sparse, and given the scarcity of clinical trials or reviews on either minimally invasive or surgical pain control options, patients are treated on a case-by-case manner. Physicians are often hesitant in performing more invasive procedures in patients with PPS give the level of complexity of consid-ering neuromuscular imbalance in the setting of joint instability and potential concom-itant arthritis.[31] Such procedures can lead to unpredictable outcomes. In addition, alteration in bone anatomy and quality, such as osteopenia and osteoporosis, make clinical decision making difficult. Steroid injections are used in patients with PPS. No clinical data support its use, and such procedures are performed in more refractory cases not responding to nonpharmacologic or conventional pharmacologic thera-pies.[19,22] There are minimal results on their efficacy but are thought to be similar to the general population receiving steroid injections for arthritic pain.[19,20] Nerve blocks have been identified in small retrospective studies as having significant improvement in joint and back pain.[32] In a study of a total of 57 patients, those who received nerve blocks with subjective average or severe pain had nearly complete relief of pain and did not require further invasive measures.[11]

Small trials and case reports have been performed on various alternative methods of pain management. Case reports have shown success in the use of intrathecal analgesic drug delivery in providing complete relief of back pain and lower limb pain.[33] Such devices have not been studied outside of case reports, and insufficient data were attributed to a lack of support for their use. A small study, though, was performed on the use of static magnetic fields on trigger points for postpolio pain. In a trial of 50 patients, those treated for PPS with trigger point static magnetic fields had a statistically significant improvement in pain.[34] Acupuncture has also been demonstrated to be efficacious in providing modest pain control in PPS. In a survey of 17 patients who received acupuncture for PPS, the average reported pain relief score on a 10-point scale was nearly 4.[11] Given its ease of implementation, safety profile, and cost-effectiveness, acupuncture can be a useful modality in PPS.

Finally, when postpolio pain is severe and refractory, surgical joint arthroplasty can be considered. Patients with PPS can present unique challenges to joint reconstruction, and surgeons must be aware of the neurologic conditions as well as the technical aspects of the surgery. Surgical approaches should be performed with the coordination of a rehabilitation team given the need for recovery of strength and motor control in the setting of a complex neuromuscular disease often with limb abnormalities. A study from the orthopedic literature demonstrated notable pain relief in all patients enrolled who underwent joint arthroplasty. There was an improvement in functional ambulation in all patients, and there was no radiographic evidence of loosening or wear of prosthesis in any patient for the entire follow-up period of 7 years.[31] Total joint arthroplasty can be safe and effective in resolving pain and improving functional status.

PROGNOSIS

Postpolo pain is not life threatening; however, its overall prognosis varies in patients. The overwhelming majority of patients with PPS experience pain at some point.[10] In a retrospective review on the impact of PPS on patients, 91% of patients reported having pain at the time of the study or within the prior 3 months.[11] Pain is a well-established common symptom in patients with PPS, noted in a variety of studies. Most patients state their pain is mild to moderate, and severe pain is less common. Pain interferes with a variety of life aspects, including work, activity, mood, sleep, and life enjoyment. The impedance of quality of life is modest; however, it still contributes to significant psychological and emotional impairment.[12,13] Demographic differences have not been identified as making any difference, although 1 study noted women to have more intense pain and for longer duration.[11,12,18]

Unlike in other neuromuscular disorders, postpolio pain syndrome is often constant without remitting periods. Patients with PPS report pain to some degree at nearly all times, and in 1 review, patients stated that since the beginning of their symptoms they had never experienced a pain-free week.[7,12] Such evidence supports the need to find multidisciplinary pain management regimens. As previously noted, a variety of lifestyle modifications and nonpharmacologic and and pharmacologic treatments are available with varying degrees of efficacy. Injections and surgery along with alternative therapies can also be used. Pain control should be tailored in individual patients. Psychosocial support is also critical in PPS, and a psychiatric referral can be helpful. An interdisciplinary approach is key in truly optimizing patients and controlling pain.[19] In addition, active patient participation in their own pain assessment is essential. Research shows patients wish to have responsibility in dealing with postpolio pain by discussing habits and life modification.[22]

Our review provides a comprehensive understanding of managing and understanding joint pain in PPS with a focus on treatment options. Pain control can be frustrating for both patients and providers, and shared management plans between patient and providers are critical in combating this syndrome. Further research is needed to truly understand and treat PPS and joint pain. At this time, a patient-tailored approach is supported in the literature with an emphasis on using multiple modalities, including nonpharmacologic and pharmacologic therapies in approaching patients.

CLINICS CARE POINTS

- Although poliovirus no longer poses the worldwide public health threat that it once did, clinicians should maintain a high index of suspicion for postpolio syndrome symptoms, particularly pain.
- It is important to evaluate the impact of pain in patients with postpolio syndrome, as it has been associated with significant reductions in quality of life.
- Pain secondary to postpolio syndrome is a clinical diagnosis; however, laboratory studies, imaging, electromyography, and nerve conduction studies or muscle biopsy may be useful to rule out other potential diagnoses.
- It is particularly important to avoid strenuous and fatiguing activity when treating pain symptoms with rehabilitation programs, as such activities may result in decreased muscle strength, fatigue, and more pain.
- When conservative management fails to control pain symptoms, alternate treatment with medications or invasive procedures may be indicated.

DISCLOSURE

The authors have nothing to disclose.

REFERENCES

1. Brown B, Oberste MS, Maher K, et al. Complete genomic sequencing shows that polioviruses and members of human enterovirus species C are closely related in the noncapsid coding region. J Virol 2003;77:8973.
2. Jane Bridges ML. Post-polio syndrome. J Consumer Health Internet 2003; 7(3):41–9.
3. LeCompte CM. Post polio syndrome: an update for the primary health care provider. Nurse Pract 1997;22(6):133–6.
4. Halstead LS. A brief history of postpolio syndrome in the United States. Arch Phys Med Rehabil 2011;92:1344–9.
5. Ramlow J, Alexander M, LaPorte R, et al. Epidemiology of the post-polio syndrome. Am J Epidemiol 1992;136:769.
6. Rekand T, Kõrv J, Farbu E, et al. Long term outcome after poliomyelitis in different health and social conditions. J Epidemiol Community Health 2003;57:368–72.
7. Jubelt B, Drucker J. Post-polio syndrome: an update. Semin Neurol 1993;13(3):283–90.
8. Dalakas M, Illa I. Post-polio syndrome: concepts in clinical diagnosis, pathogenesis, and etiology. Adv Neurol 1991;56:495.
9. Jubelt B, Cashman NR. Neurological manifestations of the post-polio syndrome. Crit Rev Neurobiol 1987;3:199.
10. Halstead LS, Rossi CD. Post-polio syndrome: results of a survey of 530 survivors. Orthopedics 1985;8:845–50.

11. Stoelb BL, Carter GT, Abresch RT, et al. Pain in persons with postpolio syndrome: frequency, intensity, and impact. Arch Phys Med Rehabil 2008;89(10):1933–40.

12. Lo JK, Robinson LR. Post-polio syndrome and the late effects of poliomyelitis: part 2. Treatment, management, and prognosis. Muscle Nerve 2018;58:760–9.

13. Widar M, Ahlström G. Experiences and consequences of pain in persons with post-polio syndrome. J Adv Nurs 1998;28:606–13.

14. Kidd D, Howard RS, Williams AJ, et al. Late functional deterioration following paralytic poliomyelitis. QJM 1997;90:189.

15. Arazpour M, Ahmadi F, Bahramizadeh M, et al. Evaluation of gait symmetry in poliomyelitis subjects: comparison of a conventional knee-ankle-foot orthosis and a new powered knee-ankle-foot orthosis. Prosthet Orthot Int 2016;40:689.

16. Farbu E, Gilhus NE, Barnes MP, et al. EFNS guideline on diagnosis and management of post-polio syndrome. Report of an EFNS Task Force. Eur J Neurol 2006; 13:795–801.

17. Jubelt B, Drucker J. In: Younger D, editor. Poliomyelitis and the post-polio syndrome in motor disorders. Philadelphia: Lippincott Williams and Wilkins; 1999. p. 381.

18. Sorenson EJ, Daube JR, Windebank A. A 15-year follow-up of neuromuscular function in patients with prior poliomyelitis. Neurology 2005;64:1070–2.

19. Koopman FS, Beelen A, Gilhus NE, et al. Treatment for postpolio syndrome. Cochrane Database Syst Rev 2015;(5):CD007818.

20. Trojan DA, Finch L. Management of post-polio syndrome. NeuroRehabilitation 1997;8(2):93–105.

21. Li H, Shing S, Chipika RH, et al. Post-polio syndrome: more than just a lower motor neuron disease. Front Neurol 2019;10:773.

22. Farbu E. Update on current and emerging treatment options for post-polio syndrome. Ther Clin Risk Manag 2010;6:307–13.

23. Waring WP, Maynard F, Grady W, et al. Influence of appropriate lower extremity orthotic management on ambulation, pain, and fatigue in a postpolio population. Arch Phys Med Rehabil 1989;70:371.

24. Jubelt B. Post-polio syndrome. Curr Treat Options Neurol 2004;6:87.

25. Elovaara I, Apostolski S, van Doorn P, et al. EFNS guidelines for the use of intravenous immunoglobulin in treatment of neurological diseases: EFNS task force on the use of intravenous immunoglobulin in treatment of neurological diseases. Eur J Neurol 2008;15(9):893–908.

26. Huang YH, Chen HC, Huang KW, et al. Intravenous immunoglobulin for postpolio syndrome: a systematic review and meta-analysis. BMC Neurol 2015;15:39.

27. Werhagen L, Borg K. Effect of intravenous immunoglobulin on pain in patients with post-polio syndrome. J Rehabil Med 2011;43:1038.

28. Bertolasi L, Frasson E, Turri M, et al. A randomized controlled trial of IV immunoglobulin in patients with postpolio syndrome. J Neurol Sci 2013;330:94.

29. Gonzalez H, Sunnerhagen KS, Sjöberg I, et al. Intravenous immunoglobulin for post-polio syndrome: a randomised controlled trial. Lancet Neurol 2006;5:493.

30. Farbu E, Rekand T, Vik-Mo E, et al. Post-polio syndrome patients treated with intravenous immunoglobulin: a double-blinded randomized controlled pilot study. Eur J Neurol 2007;14:60.

31. Hosalkar HS, Fuller DA, Rendon N, et al. Outcomes of total joint arthroplasties in adults with post-polio syndrome: results from a tertiary neuro-orthopaedic center. Curr Orthopaedic Pract 2010;21(3):273–81.

32. Lambert DA, Giannouli E, Schmidt BJ, et al. Postpolio syndrome and anesthesia. Anesthesiology 2005;103(3):638–44.

33. van Tilburg CW. Intrathecal analgesic drug delivery is effective for analgesia in a patient with post-poliomyelitis syndrome: a case report. Am J Case Rep 2016;17: 957–62.

34. Vallbona C, Hazlewood CF, Jurida G. Response of pain to static magnetic fields in postpolio patients: a double-blind pilot study. Arch Phys Med Rehabil 1997; 78(11):1200–3.

Neuromuscular Scoliosis
When, Who, Why and Outcomes

Brian D. Wishart, DO, MMS[a], Emily Kivlehan, MD[b],*

KEYWORDS

- Neuromuscular scoliosis • Neurogenic scoliosis • Orthotics • Spinal fusion
- Lower motor neuron disease

KEY POINTS

- The development of scoliosis in patients with neuromuscular disease has major impacts on function and health-related quality of life.
- Neuromuscular scoliosis classically results in a long C-shaped deformity in the coronal plane, kyphosis, and pelvic obliquity.
- The only definitive treatment to correct deformity is surgical intervention, typically with a T2-pelvic fusion.
- Optimal management consists of a multidisciplinary team, with an emphasis on goal setting and communication with caregivers and patients.

INTRODUCTION

Neuromuscular diseases have a broad clinical presentation and can affect multiple systems far beyond the nerve and muscle. Among many organ systems affected, orthopedic effects, particularly spinal deformities, have a massive impact on daily life. It has been shown that orthopedic disease that forms in a developing spine has greater long-term health, social, and mental health detriments than matched orthopedic disease that develops in adolescents and adulthood.[1] Abnormal and asymmetric muscle forces contribute to the development of scoliosis particularly in these neuromuscular patients. The presence of scoliosis is known to affect functional levels in a patient's daily care, with ambulation and sitting tolerance. It can also lead to a greater likelihood of pain, pressure ulcers, poor balance, and cardiac and respiratory complications, all of which ultimately affect how a patient interacts with the world around them.[2,3]

[a] Pediatric Physical Medicine and Rehabilitation, Spaulding Rehabilitation Hospital, Mass General Hospital for Children, 2nd Floor, 300 1st Avenue, Boston, MA 02129, USA; [b] Pediatric Physical Medicine and Rehabilitation, Spaulding Rehabilitation Hospital, Mass General Brigham, 2nd Floor, 300 1st Avenue, Boston, MA 02129, USA
* Corresponding author.
E-mail address: EJKivlehan@partners.org
Twitter: @EmilyKivlehanMD (E.K.)

Phys Med Rehabil Clin N Am 32 (2021) 547–556
https://doi.org/10.1016/j.pmr.2021.02.007
1047-9651/21/© 2021 Elsevier Inc. All rights reserved.

Poliovirus is the most common cause of epidemics of paralytic diseases.[4] In developed countries, polio is now an uncommon infectious cause of neuromuscular disease. However, despite vaccination, it has not been eradicated, with new outbreaks being seen globally.[5] During the polio epidemic, spinal deformities were seen most commonly because of asymmetric truncal paralysis causing muscle imbalance but also because of extensive symmetric paralysis involving the entire truncal musculature. Notably, a small group showed no truncal paralysis but developed scoliosis solely with limb paralysis.[6,7] The spinal deformities complicated by cardiorespiratory compromise created an urgency for innovation in scoliosis management. The classic surgical approaches at the time resulting in late complications, such as pseudoarthrosis for patients with poliomyelitis. Much of our modern scoliosis management, including orthotics such as the Milwaukee brace, and surgical treatments, including the Harrington rod, were developed during the time of the polio epidemic.[8–10]

DEFINITIONS

Spinal curvatures are described according to the anatomic plane in which the alignment deviation occurs. *Scoliosis* is dependently a multiplanar deformity defined by at least a 10° curvature in the coronal plane along with vertebral rotation in the transverse plane.[11] The coronal plane can be defined as a *dextroscoliosis* with the convexity to the right or *levoscoliosis* with the convexity to the left. Kyphosis and lordosis are descriptors of typical curvature along the sagittal plane. In the sagittal plane, a normal physiologic degree of spinal curvature is expected. An anterior concave curve in the sagittal plane is termed *kyphosis*, and a posterior concave curve is termed a *lordosis*. The cervical and lumbar spine typically shows a physiologic lordosis, whereas the thoracic spine naturally shows a kyphosis.[12] With increased lumbar lordosis, the sacral alignment in the sagittal plane can also be altered. Because of the wide variability of curvatures noted in healthy patients without spine complaints, there are not as well-defined norms noted for sagittal plane curves as there are with deviations in the coronal plane.[13]

Idiopathic scoliosis is the most common type of scoliosis and includes infantile, juvenile, and adolescent onset. Adolescent idiopathic scoliosis (AIS) is the most common within these 3 types. *Congenital scoliosis* is a scoliosis secondary to a bony congenital deformity, such as a hemivertebra. *Neuromuscular scoliosis*, the focus of this article, includes spinal deformities caused by a myopathy, or upper or lower motor neuron disease.[11,14] Typical disease processes that can lead to neuromuscular scoliosis include Duchenne muscular dystrophy, spinal muscular atrophy, cerebral palsy, Rett syndrome, spina bifida, and rare progressive neurologic diseases, such as leukodystrophies. *Scheuermann disease* is a specific abnormality noted with a kyphosis deformity in which at least 3 consecutive vertebrae are wedged at 5 or more degrees.[15] Last, syndromic, metabolic, or other causes of scoliosis can be grouped under a *miscellaneous* category of scoliosis.[11]

EPIDEMIOLOGY

Incidence of neuromuscular scoliosis in the literature is variable, depending on the underlying neuromuscular disease present. Some neuromuscular diseases have very high incidence rates: up to 90% of patients with Duchenne muscular dystrophy and 80% of patients with spinal muscular atrophy will develop scoliosis. Incidence in certain neuromuscular diseases is dependent on the area or extent of the body affected. Cerebral palsy, the most commonly seen cause of neuromuscular scoliosis, varies between 20% and 70%, which relates to the topographic distribution.[3] Mild hemiplegic patients with gross motor function classification system (GMFCS) score of 1 to 2 would be expected to have a low incidence of significant scoliosis, whereas children with spastic quadriplegic cerebral palsy and a GMFCS score of 4 to 5 would be expected to have a much higher incidence. Truncal involvement and more significant neurologic involvement are reliable predictors of scoliosis development for children with neuromuscular disease.[16] Similarly, patients with myelomeningocele demonstrate spinal involvement dependent on the level of involvement, with scoliosis incidence increasing with a higher level of myelomeningocele. In patients with myelomeningocele, 25% of those with an L5 level will develop scoliosis, whereas more than 90% of those L1 or higher will develop scoliosis.[12]

Neuromuscular scoliosis broadly includes deformities secondary to both lower motor neuron and upper motor neuron pathologic condition.[11] Polio is a disease of the alpha motor neuron, which presents a paralytic type of scoliosis because of lower motor neuron involvement. Approximately one-third of patients with poliomyelitis have been reported to develop scoliosis.[7] However, as discussed previously, this percentage is dependent on the distribution and extent of paralysis as seen in myelomeningocele. In addition, skeletally immature patients with acquired traumatic spinal cord injury and associated neurologic deficits at or above the thoracic level will go on to develop scoliosis, so it would be expected that children who develop poliomyelitis affecting the thoracic level or above will develop scoliosis.[12] As opposed to the typical S-shaped curve typically seen in adolescent idiopathic scoliosis, the most commonly seen deformity in polio-associated scoliosis is a C-shaped curve in roughly 62% of patients. The curve is most often identified in the thoracic and lumbar spine.[17,18] Lumbar curves and long C-shaped curves are known to be associated with some degree of pelvic obliquity, which will subsequently have detrimental effects on sitting balance and posture.[6,12] For wheelchair users, an inability to safely and comfortably sit has downstream effects on independence with activities daily living. Pelvic involvement will alter pressure distribution, which long term may result in ischial pain and the development of pressure wounds.[6]

PATHOPHYSIOLOGY

Neuromuscular scoliosis is caused by myopathic disease or neuropathic abnormalities and can be due to central nervous system, peripheral nervous system, or combined nerve involvement.[15] Weakness and paralysis, as seen in polio and other neuromuscular diseases, as well as poor muscular control and potentially spasticity interfere with the balanced muscular forces on the spine. This muscular imbalance can result in an inability to symmetrically maintain the spine under the force of gravity. During rapid skeletal growth, these imbalances can be exacerbated, resulting in rapidly progressive curves. Truncal weakness in neuromuscular patients causes them to collapse into a kyphosis, resulting in a high incidence of kyphotic deformities. In AIS, the curve is expected to stop progressing after skeletal maturity. In significant contrast, neuromuscular scoliosis, and seen particularly in polio scoliosis, curves continue to progress after skeletal maturity.[7]

There are multiple risk factors for ongoing and rapid progression of a spinal deformity in neuromuscular patients. With increased neurologic involvement and more severe muscular imbalance, there is a more significant risk for progression. Prolonged abnormal posture results in asymmetric forces on the vertebral growth plates, which can cause a cycle of further and progressive curve development.[19] Compared with spasticity, the presence of weakness may be more likely to contribute to ongoing progression, as patients with cerebral palsy do not see a difference in progression rates between patients with intrathecal baclofen pumps and those without intrathecal baclofen.[20] More severe curves are more likely to have more rapid progression particularly after they develop a Cobb angel of 50°. Rapid growth, such as during the pubertal growth spurt, or progressive weakness can cause progression as well.[15]

DIAGNOSTICS

Screening for scoliosis is typically performed with the Adams forward bend test with the use of a "scoliometer." In this examination, the patient stands with feet approximately 15 cm apart, flexes at the trunk with knees straight, shoulders and arms hanging loose. The examiner observes the patient from behind and focuses on 3 areas, the thoracic, thoracolumbar, and lumbar regions.[21] The Adams test has been said to identify asymmetry of the rib cage caused by vertebral rotation.[22] It is most reliable in older children.[21] The scoliometer is normally used at the thoracic, thoracolumbar, and lumbar regions, and any measurement greater than 0° is defined as abnormal, and greater than 7° should be referred. The angle measured with the scoliometer does not correspond to that measured in radiographs.[21]

Posterioanterior (PA) and lateral radiographs are the imaging modality of choice for scoliosis.[23] To assess the true effects of gravity on the spine, weight-bearing films while standing are ideal.

For patients who are nonambulatory, weight-bearing in a seated position can be alternatively used.[12] As this can be challenging to obtain, supine PA and lateral films can be used but are not ideal. If supine films are taken, bending and traction films should be considered.[7] Lower-radiation radiographs are now available and should be used if possible for serial examinations. Once radiographs are performed, Cobb angles and Risser index can be calculated and monitored with repeat radiographs.

More advanced imaging is indicated in several instances. Computed tomography scans can be used for surgical planning, for evaluation of congenital bony abnormalities, and for concerns for a suspected tumor cause. MRI is indicated for patients with early-onset scoliosis. Abnormal progression, pain, and surgical planning are also indications for MRI. Despite these indications, MRI is not typically obtained in neuromuscular scoliosis patients.[24]

Cobb Angle

Definition: Degree of curvature in the coronal plane.

Limitations: Only assesses a single plane, the coronal plane, of a multiplanar deformity. The severity of the curve is linearly associated with the measured Cobb angle.

To measure:

1. Identify the most tilted superior and inferior vertebrae of the curve.
2. Draw a line parallel to the upper end plate of the most superior tilted vertebra above the apex of the curve, and another line parallel to the lower end plate of the most inferior tilted vertebra below the apex of the curve.
3. The intersection of these 2 lines is the Cobb angle. Classically, a perpendicular line can be drawn to these lines, and the intersection of these lines can be measured. With computer imaging software, this angle can now be measured digitally.[25]

Risser Index

Definition: A scale of skeletal maturity, graded from 0 to 5 by dividing migration of apophysis into quarters. The iliac apophysis is more easily visualized than the vertebral growth plates, and the completion skeletal maturity is simultaneous for the iliac apophysis and vertebral growth plates. As such, the iliac apophysis as it migrates posteromedially toward the sacrum is monitored.[26]

Limitations: Stage 0 and stage 5 look similar and may be confused.

To measure:

0: No ossification of the apophysis identified.
1: Apophysis present, but less than 25% of iliac crest.
2: Apophysis is 25% to 50% of iliac crest.
3: Apophysis is 50% to 75% of iliac crest.
4: Apophysis is 75% to 100% of iliac crest.
5: Apophysis has completed fusion.[27]

MANAGEMENT
Treatment

Management of scoliosis should be considered on a spectrum, ideally starting with more conservative approaches and increasing to more invasive approaches as warranted. If identified early, patients are observed with regular radiographic follow-up.[6] Observation can be continued for patients with curves less than 25° and should be watched for curve progression. Much of the evidence for this comes from patients with idiopathic scoliosis, and it should be noted there are significant differences when caring for neuromuscular scoliosis. Typically, patients are monitored every 3 to 6 months with repeat films. Films should be obtained sooner, every 3 months, if there are concerns for rapid progression or if the patient is younger and more skeletally immature.[7] Although different causes of neuromuscular scoliosis are often considered together, each patient's underlying neuromuscular condition must be taken into account when evaluating and determining a treatment plan.

There have been certain therapies and scoliosis-specific exercises developed to be used during this observation period with variable outcomes. Proper equipment, positioning, and orthotics can ideally allow for optimal function and comfort. Within the neuromuscular world, Duchenne muscular dystrophy is unique in having a medical treatment with steroids that can slow the progression of scoliosis and potentially eliminate the need for surgery.[28] In clinical practice, these interventions are not always done in a stepwise fashion and often overlap.

Therapies

Physical therapy referral can allow for stretching to maintain range of motion, helping to prevent contractures, maintain chest wall mobility, and assess for equipment needs.[3] Physical therapy and other manual therapies may be beneficial for pain management as well. Scoliosis-specific exercises are most often used for AIS, although available evidence is variable, partially because of the variable natural progression of AIS itself. There are multiple schools regarding conservative management of idiopathic scoliosis. There is evidence for some effectiveness in AIS with these different therapies, although the applicability to neuromuscular scoliosis remains unclear. One case report has demonstrated effectiveness with the Schroth method, a scoliosis-specific exercise program, for a patient with scoliosis secondary to polio.[29] However, more evidence is needed. One benefit that has been emphasized by families is the ability to gain some control over the disease process.[30] With education and expectation setting, these therapeutic approaches would be low risk in causing any harm.

The following schools of therapy have been described in use for scoliosis[30,31]:

- Lyon approach from France

- Katharina Schroth Asklepios approach from Germany
- Scientific Exercise Approach to Scoliosis from Italy
- Barcelona Scoliosis Physical Therapy School approach from Spain
- DoboMed approach from Poland
- Side shift approach from the United Kingdom
- Functional individual therapy of scoliosis approach from Poland

Bracing

Bracing is a key component in the management of idiopathic scoliosis. It has been shown to slow progression and decrease the need for surgical intervention. In AIS, there is a dose response to bracing; with increased hours per day worn, there is an increased likelihood of halting the curve.[32] The use of bracing in neuromuscular scoliosis is done with different goals. It can be useful to help with positioning, improve posture, sitting balance, and function as well as comfort but has been shown to have little effect on the progression of the scoliotic curve.[2,27] Unlike the response to bracing in AIS, bracing generally does not halt progression of curvature in neuromuscular scoliosis.[12,33,34]

Bracing in neuromuscular patients should focus on function and maximizing quality of life. The balance between corrective forces and accommodating for the deformity needs to be thoughtfully addressed. To address the curvature, general bracing principle of providing balanced forces must be applied, to create a bending moment at curve vertex. In order to do this, a 3-pressure-point model is used with 1 point over the apex of the convexity and 2 points above and below the apex on the concavity of the curve. There are several types of braces that are used for the management of scoliosis:

- Milwaukee: Cervicothoracolumbo-sacral orthosis
- Wilmington: Thoracolumbosacral orthosis (TLSO) custom fitted off a cast taken of patient.
- Boston: TLSO constructed from a prefabricated symmetric module with no metal rods.
- Suspension Trunk Orthosis: TLSO, which does not rest on the patient's pelvis but instead directly on seat and has been described specifically for neuromuscular patients.[35]

Experienced and thoughtful therapists are an invaluable part of the treatment team to assist with appropriate evaluations for equipment needs. Custom seating options and adjustments to a patient's wheelchair can help to maximize function and assist with comfort. For example, wheelchairs can be adjusted to include lateral supports and provide appropriate offloading of pressure points.

For cases in which cardiorespiratory function is compromised, effects of the brace on the respiratory system must be considered. For patients with severe scoliosis and effective curve correction by a brace, respiratory parameters can be altered.[36] Soft braces may be sufficient to improve posture and balance, with better tolerance.[37] Brace design must not impede the use of accessory respiratory musculature or chest excursion for patients who require this for adequate ventilation.

SURGERY

In AIS, there are well-accepted surgical criteria, with surgery typically occurring after the curve has progressed beyond 40°. In neuromuscular scoliosis, medical fragility causes the decision to pursue surgery to be much less straightforward.[34] In addition to the Cobb angle, respiratory status, curve flexibility or rigidity, and pelvic obliquity are all additional factors. Complications of corrective surgery in neuromuscular scoliosis are much higher than with AIS. The most common complication is neurologic injury. Scoliosis surgery is known to have detrimental effects on pulmonary function testing regardless of cause, so the risk of respiratory deterioration for children who already have pulmonary disease must be considered.[38] Complications have been found to be higher when surgery is performed before 13 years of age.[39] Still, after surgery, there are reported improvements in pain, self-image, and function.[40] Complication rate can be close to 80% with the most common complications reported being

- Pulmonary
- Implant failure (ie, rod breakage)
- Infection
- Neurologic
- Pseudarthrosis

The classic fusion level is from T2 through the pelvis.[3,11] Pelvic extension is needed because of the associated pelvic deformities and obliquity in neuromuscular scoliosis.[12] Postoperative care is complicated by precautions, including limited hip flexion and spinal rotation. Equipment to assist with transfers will be needed during this time. In addition, prior equipment likely will need to be adjusted given postoperative changes in posture and pressure distribution.[41] Admissions to inpatient rehabilitation should be considered during this time. Intensive rehabilitation allows for close monitoring and prevention of pressure wounds, maintenance of range of motion, reconditioning, optimization of nutrition, wound monitoring, pain management, bowel and bladder management, assessment of new equipment needs, or current equipment adjustments, with daily medical physician oversight.[3] Families should be educated that it may take an extended time period, sometimes from 6 months to a year, until the child has returned to baseline level of function.

OUTCOMES

Outcomes in neuromuscular scoliosis are variable, even for the most definitive treatment available. Management plans require a multidisciplinary team, with shared decision making with families and caregivers. Education is a key component, especially for families to know that curves are likely to progress despite therapy, positioning, and bracing. Expectation setting and shared goal setting should be a key component. Surgery, regardless of the degree of curve correction, consistently does improve quality-of-life scores.[42,43]

CLINICS CARE POINTS

- Scoliosis is seen in most patients with neuromuscular disease involving the truncal musculature.
- Rapid progression can be seen through adolescents and ongoing progression into adulthood.
- Bracing is typically unsuccessful in halting the progression of neuromuscular scoliosis.
- Surgical techniques have improved, although neuromuscular patients continue to have high rates of complications following fusion.
- Shared goal setting and realistic expectations are needed before surgical intervention.

DISCLOSURE

The authors have nothing to disclose.

REFERENCES

1. Shavelle RM, Devivo MJ, Paculdo DR, et al. Long-term survival after childhood spinal cord injury. J Spinal Cord Med 2007;30(Suppl 1):S48–54.
2. Majd ME, Muldowny DS, Holt RT. Natural history of scoliosis in the institutionalized adult cerebral palsy population. Spine (Phila Pa 1976) 1997;22(13):1461–6.
3. Roberts SB, Tsirikos AI. Factors influencing the evaluation and management of neuromuscular scoliosis: a review of the literature. J Back Musculoskelet Rehabil 2016;29(4):613–23.
4. Marx A, Glass JD, Sutter RW. Differential diagnosis of acute flaccid paralysis and its role in poliomyelitis surveillance. Epidemiol Rev 2000;22(2):298–316.
5. Chard AN, Datta SD, Tallis G, et al. Progress toward polio eradication — worldwide, January 2018–March 2020. MMWR Morb Mortal Wkly Rep 2020;69:784–9.
6. Leong JC, Wilding K, Mok CK, et al. Surgical treatment of scoliosis following poliomyelitis. A review of one hundred and ten cases. J Bone Joint Surg Am 1981;63(5):726–40.
7. Colonna P. A study of paralytic scoliosis based on five hundred cases of poliomyelitis. J Bone Joint Surg Am 1941;23:335–53.
8. Desai SK, Brayton A, Chua VB, et al. The lasting legacy of Paul Randall Harrington to pediatric spine surgery: historical vignette. J Neurosurg Spine 2013;18(2):170–7.
9. Harrington PR. The history and development of Harrington instrumentation. Clin Orthop Relat Res 1973;(93):110–2.
10. Blount WP, Schmidt AC, Keever ED, et al. The Milwaukee brace in the operative treatment of scoliosis. J Bone Joint Surg Am 1958;40-A(3):511–25.
11. El-Hawary R, Chukwunyerenwa C. Update on evaluation and treatment of scoliosis. Pediatr Clin North Am 2014;61(6):1223–41.
12. Berven S, Bradford DS. Neuromuscular scoliosis: causes of deformity and principles for evaluation and management. Semin Neurol 2002;22(2):167–78.
13. Stagnara P, De Mauroy JC, Dran G, et al. Reciprocal angulation of vertebral bodies in a sagittal plane: approach to references for the evaluation of kyphosis and lordosis. Spine (Phila Pa 1976) 1982;7(4):335–42.
14. Vialle R, Thevenin-Lemoine C, Mary P. Neuromuscular scoliosis. Orthop Traumatol Surg Res 2013;99(1 Suppl):S124–39.
15. Wenger DR, Frick SL. Scheuermann kyphosis. Spine (Phila Pa 1976) 1999;24(24):2630–9.
16. Bertoncelli CM, Bertoncelli D, Elbaum L, et al. Validation of a clinical prediction model for the development of neuromuscular scoliosis: a multinational study. Pediatr Neurol 2018;79:14–20.
17. Baliga S, McMillan T, Sutherland A, et al. The prevalence and severity of joint problems and disability in patients with poliomyelitis in Urban India. Open Orthop J 2015;9:204–9.
18. Mayer PJ, Dove J, Ditmanson M, et al. Post-poliomyelitis paralytic scoliosis. A review of curve patterns and results of surgical treatments in 118 consecutive patients. Spine (Phila Pa 1976) 1981;6(6):573–82.
19. McCarthy RE. Management of neuromuscular scoliosis. Orthop Clin North Am 1999;30(3):435–49, viii.

20. Shilt JS, Lai LP, Cabrera MN, et al. The impact of intrathecal baclofen on the natural history of scoliosis in cerebral palsy. J Pediatr Orthop 2008;28(6):684–7.
21. Patias P, Grivas TB, Kaspiris A, et al. A review of the trunk surface metrics used as scoliosis and other deformities evaluation indices. Scoliosis 2010;5:12.
22. Bunnell WP. An objective criterion for scoliosis screening. J Bone Joint Surg Am 1984;66(9):1381–7.
23. Jones JY, Saigal G, Palasis S, et al. ACR Appropriateness Criteria((R)) Scoliosis-Child. J Am Coll Radiol 2019;16(5S):S244–51.
24. Halawi MJ, Lark RK, Fitch RD. Neuromuscular scoliosis: current concepts. Orthopedics 2015;38(6):e452–6.
25. Cobb JR. Outline for the study of scoliosis. Am Acad Orthop Surg Instr Course Lect 1948;5:261–75.
26. Risser JC. The classic: the iliac apophysis: an invaluable sign in the management of scoliosis. 1958. Clin Orthop Relat Res 2010;468(3):643–53.
27. Hacquebord JH, Leopold SS. In brief: the Risser classification: a classic tool for the clinician treating adolescent idiopathic scoliosis. Clin Orthop Relat Res 2012; 470(8):2335–8.
28. Lebel DE, Corston JA, McAdam LC, et al. Glucocorticoid treatment for the prevention of scoliosis in children with Duchenne muscular dystrophy: long-term follow-up. J Bone Joint Surg Am 2013;95(12):1057–61.
29. Torres B. Katharina Schroth method for treatment of post-polio scoliosis in an adult. Scoliosis 2007;2(S1):1.
30. Berdishevsky H, Lebel VA, Bettany-Saltikov J, et al. Physiotherapy scoliosis-specific exercises - a comprehensive review of seven major schools. Scoliosis Spinal Disord 2016;11:20.
31. Negrini S, Aulisa AG, Aulisa L, et al. 2011 SOSORT guidelines: orthopaedic and rehabilitation treatment of idiopathic scoliosis during growth. Scoliosis 2012; 7(1):3.
32. Weinstein SL, Dolan LA, Wright JG, et al. Effects of bracing in adolescents with idiopathic scoliosis. N Engl J Med 2013;369(16):1512–21.
33. Tsirikos AI, Smith G. Scoliosis in patients with Friedreich's ataxia. J Bone Joint Surg Br 2012;94(5):684–9.
34. Sarwark J, Sarwahi V. New strategies and decision making in the management of neuromuscular scoliosis. Orthop Clin North Am 2007;38(4):485–96, v.
35. Kotwicki T, Durmala J, Czubak J. Bracing for neuromuscular scoliosis: orthosis construction to improve the patient's function. Disabil Rehabil Assist Technol 2008;3(3):161–9.
36. Noble-Jamieson CM, Heckmatt JZ, Dubowitz V, et al. Effects of posture and spinal bracing on respiratory function in neuromuscular disease. Arch Dis Child 1986;61(2):178–81.
37. Letts M, Rathbone D, Yamashita T, et al. Soft Boston orthosis in management of neuromuscular scoliosis: a preliminary report. J Pediatr Orthop 1992;12(4):470–4.
38. Yuan N, Fraire JA, Margetis MM, et al. The effect of scoliosis surgery on lung function in the immediate postoperative period. Spine (Phila Pa 1976) 2005; 30(19):2182–5.
39. Sharma S, Wu C, Andersen T, et al. Prevalence of complications in neuromuscular scoliosis surgery: a literature meta-analysis from the past 15 years. Eur Spine J 2013;22(6):1230–49.
40. Godzik J, Lenke LG, Holekamp T, et al. Complications and outcomes of complex spine reconstructions in poliomyelitis-associated spinal deformities: a single-institution experience. Spine (Phila Pa 1976) 2014;39(15):1211–6.

41. Mullender M, Blom N, De Kleuver M, et al. A Dutch guideline for the treatment of scoliosis in neuromuscular disorders. Scoliosis 2008;3:14.

42. Brooks JT, Sponseller PD. What's new in the management of neuromuscular scoliosis. J Pediatr Orthop 2016;36(6):627–33.

43. Bohtz C, Meyer-Heim A, Min K. Changes in health-related quality of life after spinal fusion and scoliosis correction in patients with cerebral palsy. J Pediatr Orthop 2011;31(6):668–73.

Psychiatric Approaches and Outcomes

Stephanie T. Machell, PsyD[a,b],*

KEYWORDS

- Post-polio syndrome • Psychotherapy • Medical trauma

KEY POINTS

- Although polio survivors benefit from addressing the energy drain created by unresolved mental health issues, their psychological needs often are overlooked.
- Polio-informed psychological treatment and medical treatment informed by the survivor's psychological needs enable patients to address polio within a whole-life context.
- By providing empathic support for their patients' mental health needs, physicians and other medical providers can create a culture of mental health within the polio clinic.

INTRODUCTION

...[T]he virus of poliomyelitis is not the patient's sole enemy... He has the enemy of fear, he has the enemy of uncertainty about the future, he has the enemy of worry caused by his disturbance over his illness and what it is going to do to his parents and his relationships with his friends. ...[T]hey must fight the enemy on all fronts. To fight him on the physical front alone and leave the patient vulnerable to psychological destruction is to lose the war.

—*Morton Seidenfeld[1]*

In 1946, Morton Seidenfeld was appointed director of psychological services for the National Federation for Infantile Paralysis (NFIP). He believed that once polio's acute phase ended, 75% to 90% of a patient's needs had a psychological component that should be addressed by making psychological services an integral part of the care provided.[1] Despite his advocacy (seen as newsworthy enough to be reported by *The New York Times*[2]), his vision never was realized. Few polio rehabilitation programs included mental health professionals. The vast majority of those that included mental health facets provided only the most cursory services. Seidenfeld's 1952 survey of the polio literature showed that less than 2% focused on psychological needs.[1]

Based on the negative memories of interactions with mental health professionals reported in polio survivors' memoirs,[3,4] it may be just as well. Mid–twentieth century

a Independent Practice, Belmont, MA, USA; b Independent Practice, Framingham, MA, USA
* 30 Churchill Street, Saugus, MA 01906.
E-mail address: drstm@mindspring.com

Phys Med Rehabil Clin N Am 32 (2021) 557–568
https://doi.org/10.1016/j.pmr.2021.03.002
1047-9651/21/© 2021 Elsevier Inc. All rights reserved.
pmr.theclinics.com

psychotherapy's psychoanalytic framework was ill suited to address issues related to medical trauma or disability. The few pioneers in the new specialty of rehabilitation psychology subscribed to what had been referred to as the "polio zeitgeist,"[5] guiding patients toward a form of emotional, social, and cognitive "adjustment" analogous to the physical and occupational therapist's efforts to make polio bodies acceptable to the cultural surround they would need to inhabit in order to succeed.

And succeed they did, becoming the best educated, highest achieving, and most frequently married of all people with disabilities. This success came at a high price, exacting a physical toll in the form of post-polio syndrome (PPS). As Seidenfeld predicted, it exacted a psychological toll as well. In the postwar era, when the specialty of rehabilitation psychology was coming into being, providing psychological services in general hospitals and rehabilitation units was a radical idea. Now, although it is common to find mental health professionals providing care in rehabilitation settings, accessing polio-informed mental health care remains challenging due to lack of information and awareness about polio and the number of polio survivors in the population at large.

The goal of this article is to help those already working with this population, in particular medical providers, infuse psychological principles into their work. Providers ought to know how to find and integrate mental health professionals into their teams and/or make appropriate community referrals. Mental health professionals currently working with polio survivors must consider ways of expanding this work and encourage those trained in working with chronic illness, physical disability, and psychological trauma to develop an interest in joining their ranks. After a brief review of the literature, discussions around the psychological issues polio survivors face, the provision of polio-informed mental health treatment, and ways providers and clinics can address mental health issues that may arise during medical treatment. Finally, this article explores future directions for providing polio-informed mental health services, including the promise of telehealth to expand such services and the need to train the next generation of providers.

A word about terminology. For the purposes of the article, 'polio survivor' is used to refer to any individual with a history of polio. *Mental health professional* or *psychotherapist* is used if a specialty (eg, psychiatry, psychology, social work, or licensed counseling) is irrelevant. *Provider* generically refers to any provider, including mental health professionals.

HISTORY

Although the psychological effects of polio were noted in articles written in the 1930s, the NFIP did not fund psychological research or treatment until the 1940s.[1] As discussed previously, both remained inadequate. Psychological services often were limited to assessment of educational and/or vocational needs,[6] although some papers[7,8] provide models for more expansive services. Some researchers and clinicians[5,9] address adjustment issues after acute polio, contradicting the accepted paradigm that only those with preexisting mental pathology would be affected by the polio experience.

The pressure for adjustment to disability had the potential to cause a survivor to create an outwardly conforming "bifurcated" self.[10] PPS often resulted in the unraveling of this self. Research into the effects of PPS on psychological functioning[11] found that survivors often began to remember their original polio experiences and the concomitant distress they had felt. Other researchers[12-14] report that those with PPS had increased levels of symptoms, including anxiety, irritability, and depression, although some studies[15,16] report that most polio survivors functioned well in spite of this, even thriving and finding ways of making meaning.

Some researchers and clinicians believe that this ability to function well is due to the patterns of coping common to polio survivors. Many, if not most, can be categorized as hard-driving achievers, a style inculcated into them in rehabilitation and reinforced by role models like Franklin Roosevelt.[11,16,17] For them, letting go of the polio zeitgeist,[5] that hard work results in triumph over polio,[17] and the emphasis on walking regardless of the costs involved[1] pose a great challenge to dealing with PPS. Maynard and Roller[18] posit that polio survivors fall into 2 groups based on how they related to and coped with polio (**Table 1**).

Little has been written about psychotherapy with polio survivors or how medical providers can address their psychological needs. Early articles note but do not elaborate on use of a stage model of grieving and accepting disability.[19,20] Bruno and Frick[11] recommend treatment aimed at changing a type A personality and accepting disability but note that their patients frequently relapse. Cognitive behavior therapy has been reported to be helpful for helping patients learn skills for coping with and accepting disability.[21] Some investigators[22,23] suggest narrative approaches help integrate the polio story. Because so many polio survivors have experienced psychological trauma, trauma-informed treatment is recommended strongly by several investigators regardless of whether the survivor meets full criteria for posttraumatic stress

Table 1		
Coping styles of polio survivors		
Passers	**Minimizers**	**Identifiers**
"Passed" as nondisabled in most situations	More visibly disabled, often used assistive devices (crutches and/or bracing) throughout lifetime	Have incorporated disability into identity
Disability ranges from invisible to patient believing it is	Place considerable value on "overcoming" disability. Identity issues may focus on what it means to no longer be able to do so.	May be acutely distressed by loss of abilities given how little they have
Highest level of distress over PPS	May have more visible deformity	Although they are accustomed to using assistive devices and supports, they may grieve loss of abilities and independence and fear real consequences these might have for them.
Difference between pre-PPS and post-PPS functioning perceived as profound	Least disabled of this group viewed may have viewed themselves as "passers"	
Often experience central fatigue as their most prominent symptom		
Frequently struggle with identity issues		
Resistant to use of assistive devices		

disorder (PTSD).[1,22–25] Bieniek and Kennedy[26] provide helpful recommendations for polio survivors interested in pursuing psychotherapy. Many polio memoirs[3,4,26] describe successful courses of treatment and subsequent improvements in functioning and quality of life.

NATURE OF THE PROBLEM

Polio survivors are a heterogenous group united by their encounter with the poliovirus. How it affected them involves a complex interplay between their own constitutional makeup (including their age and which life tasks were interrupted by their illness), their family, and their cultural surround; the physical effects of the virus on their bodies; and their subjective experience of illness and recovery.

Although different, their experiences during the acute phase and rehabilitation had much in common, as did their lives afterward. Those unable to pass as able-bodied experienced stigma related to others' perception of and attitudes toward people with disabilities, discrimination in various circumstances, and lack of accessibility. Especially for those who had polio as toddlers, attachment issues can lead to separation anxiety or detachment from significant others. Insistence on independence can alienate others or confuse them when PPS leads to new requests for help. Anxiety and perfectionism can result in excessive need to control others and the environment. PPS can prevent a survivor from engaging in activities with family and friends, who may not understand or believe that exercise could possibly lead to weakness.

The coping styles identified by Maynard and Roller[18] led to particular issues (see **Table 1**). Passers and minimizers may experience more issues around changed identity as they struggle with seeing themselves as having a disability, perhaps for the first time, whereas identifiers may fear losing hard-won independence.

Box 1 contains a list of psychological issues frequently faced by polio survivors. It is important to remember that *issues* is not synonymous with *pathology*. Although all polio survivors grapple with some issues related to their experience of polio and/or PPS, a vast majority do not meet diagnostic criteria for a mental health disorder as defined by the *Diagnostic and Statistical Manual of Mental Disorders* (Fifth Edition) or the *International Classification of Diseases, Tenth Revision*. Those who do meet criteria most often have what is referred to as an adjustment disorder, defined as emotional or behavioral symptoms related to specific stressors. Some survivors may have what might be called *shadow syndromes*, for example, symptoms that do not fully meet criteria for diagnosing a specific disorder.

In my practice, the most common of these disorders is PTSD. A patient may have mild or severe but transient and recurrent symptoms, often in response to triggering stimuli. Because much of the trauma experienced by polio survivors could be categorized as medical trauma (**Box 2**), such triggering often occurs in medical settings, which subsequently are avoided with problematic results. The survivor may have difficulty trusting medical providers who at best have little understanding of polio and at worst may invalidate PPS or provide frightening, even damaging, misdiagnoses. Developing PPS also can revive trauma-related memories.

Not all trauma leads to PTSD. The polio experience, however, creates conditions that favor its development. Polio survivors who developed PTSD may have had other traumatic experiences that contributed to the development of the condition, though the medical trauma of the polio experience can be sufficient cause in itself, especially when combined with the cumulative, small *t*, traumas (now referred to as microaggressions or, as 1 patient observed, "Death by a thousand cuts") that people with disabilities incur throughout a lifetime.

Box 1
Psychological issues that may affect polio survivors
Separation/attachment issues; fear of abandonment
Feelings of detachment from environment, self, and others
Body image, shame and "internalized cripophobia"/stigma/discrimination
Identity/self-image related to PPS
Claustrophobia
Amnesia for part or all of the polio experience (other than lack of recall due to age or medical status)
Anxiety or dissociation when exposed to stimuli reminiscent of polio experience
Trust issues (with medical providers or others)
Perfectionism, striving, extreme drive to succeed (type A personality)
Adjustment to/acceptance of new/increased disability, accepting assistive devices
Ambivalence about accepting help/feelings of uselessness/becoming a burden
Lack of empathy from family/significant others
Grief related to loss of ability/role/functioning
Social isolation
Depression
Anxiety/panic attacks
PTSD (full syndrome or shadow syndrome), including medical trauma (see **Box 2**)

THERAPEUTIC OPTIONS

As discussed previously, polio survivors are a heterogenous group. As such, they can and do experience a full range of medical and psychiatric issues. Polio is not the whole of who they are. But like a golden thread in a tapestry, it is shot through the fabric of their being. When working with polio survivors, it is critical to follow this thread and address the ways it has interacted with other life experiences, practicing what might be called polio-informed mental health care.

For any new patient, engagement with the mental health provider begins before the first contact by phone or in the waiting room. A warm handoff in a clinic context, a strong recommendation from a trusted provider or peer, reading a column or hearing a talk, and observing the clinician interacting with others all build trust and increase the likelihood that patients will keep their first appointment.

Although some patients know what they want out of the consultation, others are uncertain what a mental health provider can offer. For them, providing a menu of options of what the patient might address can be helpful (**Box 3**). With both groups, including a more or less oblique reference to the possibility that polio and/or PPS could be traumatic is meant to serve notice that the provider is open to hearing difficult things should the patient wish to address them. Conducting a structured psychiatric interview provides less information at times. Those who have symptoms eventually disclose or manifest them.

The focus of the initial consultation may be on psychoeducation about mental health issues common to polio survivors, including considering the need for and the potential risks and benefits of ongoing treatment. The focus may be on the shock of receiving a

---

Box 2
Examples of medical trauma experienced by polio survivors

- Acute polio experience (including isolation, lack of understanding/explanation, life-threatening/changing illness, paralysis/helplessness, iron lung, hyperesthesia, high fever)
- Waking up during surgery
- Repeated surgeries/hospitalizations
- Abuse in hospital/rehabilitation and/or by subsequent providers
- Cumulative trauma/microaggressions by medical providers
- Misdiagnoses, including failure to diagnose PPS
- Witnessing deaths in hospital/rehabilitation

---

definitive PPS diagnosis, the implications for themselves and their families, and/or ambivalence about the life changes (including recommendations for reducing or leaving work or accepting new assistive devices) or the ways being in the polio clinic stimulates traumatic memories. It may focus on concrete questions about accessing services, applying for Social Security Disability Insurance (SSDI) or long-term disability, or whether to downsize or move into more accessible housing. It might focus on issues around energy conservation or pacing. It even could be on issues completely unrelated to polio.

For many patients, the initial consultation is all they need. Having their questions answered and/or fears allayed may be sufficient. Others, because of distance or other barriers, may wish to but be unable to follow-up. Open communication and the possibility of returning on subsequent visits to the clinic and/or contacting for further consultation for themselves, family members, or their own psychotherapists are helpful.

Many patients return annually for follow-up. The psychotherapeutic work with polio survivors starts from the belief that each individual has a unique blend of affective, cognitive, behavioral, physiologic, and social issues deriving from the interaction of heredity and environment. Although everyone is different, commonalities are shared

---

Box 3
Issues that may be the focus of polio-informed mental health consultation or treatment

Feelings/issues stimulated by coming to polio clinic

Coping with/adjusting to PPS diagnosis

Explaining diagnosis to family/significant others, enlisting help versus maintaining independence

Resistance to need to change behavior or lifestyle, including need for assistive devices

Skills training for energy conservation/pacing

Applying for services/SSDI/long-term disability

Issues around accessibility/accommodation

Body image/shame/internalized cripophobia

Grief

Psychological/medical trauma

---

due to these same factors. Using an integrative relational framework means interventions can be tailored to address particular needs. With a given polio survivor in any given session, various techniques may be implemented. For example, cognitive behavior techniques might be used to address issues related to energy conservation or pacing, improving sleep, adjusting to using assistive devices, or reducing symptoms of anxiety or depression. Existential techniques might be used to address grief over loss of role or functioning or of identity and to make meaning of the polio experience. Trauma-informed, insight-oriented techniques might be used to process experiences or memories and to help patients understand how these continue to affect them in the present as well as to address issues regarding attachment. Mind-body techniques could be used in combination with the aforementioned treatments to process trauma, cope with pain or fatigue, or even reduce anxiety.

As with any patient, frequency and length of the treatment episode vary with need and personal preference. Many patients choose to reduce frequency or return as needed. To facilitate this, open door terminations should be provided, encouraging patients to return or be in touch as needed.

Many polio survivors have had 1 or more negative experiences with medical providers, ranging from cumulative microaggressions to outright physical and sexual abuse. Providers lacking knowledge of polio may have misdiagnosed the patient in damaging, often frightening, ways. Trust issues often cause survivors to resist, even avoid, medical treatment. Although finding a place where polio is "spoken" can make survivors feel comforted and understood, it can also can be anxiety-provoking. A definitive PPS diagnosis is life altering for patients, often throwing into question everything that previously helped them overcome polio. Discussions of energy conservation, giving up valued activities and roles, and the need to accept help and assistive devices stir up fears about the future. Certain parts of the evaluation, such as a brace clinic, may trigger painful, even traumatic, memories.

Understanding the psychological issues involved can make the difference between treatment resistance and compliance. Just as mental health professionals working in rehabilitation settings need basic working knowledge of their patients' physical conditions, medical professionals need basic working knowledge of their psychological issues (see **Boxes 1** and **2**). Often medical providers are reluctant to address mental health out of fear that they will say or do something to damage a patient, although not doing so may be more damaging. In addition to reducing trust and reinforcing stigma, addressing mental health issues as part of medical treatment conveys the message that the mind is indeed separate from the body and that psychological concerns are irrelevant to medical treatment. Patients may become more reticent about their reality and fail to provide information that would facilitate treatment.

Incorporating psychological issues into medical care does not mean a provider should provide mental health treatment outside the scope of training. All patients may need is for their concerns to be heard. Empathic listening and reassurance often are enough. Many of the issues that polio survivors discuss in psychological treatment can be addressed by medical providers as well (eg, physical and occupational therapists may provide skills training in energy conservation; physicians can address anxiety about future functioning and the need to plan for changes in this; and all can address concerns about assistive device use and how to communicate with family members).

Admitting the issues presented are beyond a provider's scope and making a referral is appropriate too and far more likely to be accepted when a patient feels understood. When making referrals to mental health professionals, it is important to be clear about why this is being done. Unfortunately, stigma about mental health treatment still exists. Survivors who have encountered physicians and others skeptical about PPS may have been told the condition was "all in their minds." A mental health referral made with no explanation of the benefits of such treatment of polio survivors can make them feel their concerns are being minimized or that the provider thinks they are "crazy." A strategy to reassure is telling them that far from being "all in their mind," the condition is "all in their body"—but because of the mind-body connection, treating their minds will help their bodies function better.

Ideally that referral will be to a mental health professional who is part of the rehabilitation team. When, as is often the case, there are no mental health providers available experienced in working with polio survivors, referrals to those specializing in rehabilitation or health psychology, psychological (in particular medical) trauma, geropsychology, or grief may be appropriate, especially when providers have taken the time to get to know them and their approach.

Although having a mental health professional on the rehabilitation team is ideal, where institutional or financial issues prevent this, the team still can create a clinic-wide culture of mental health that begins with the sensitivity shown by the intake person to hesitation and questions that a patient may have, extends to the receptionist's compassionate attitude toward possible apprehensions on the first day of the evaluation, and then extends to the care and empathic listening of every provider the patient subsequently sees and the implied warm handoff to a trusted mental health professional in the community. Patients who reject such referrals at the time of the evaluation may benefit from the inclusion in clinic information packets of materials related to mental health and polio, allowing them to consider options for help if issues arise afterward.

CLINICAL OUTCOMES

Consistent with the professional literature and polio narratives, cited previously, some polio survivors report psychotherapy as helpful. Specific factors endorsed as helpful are the opportunity to talk openly about their polio experiences with an empathic other; psychoeducation that normalizes their social-emotional experiences; learning specific coping skills, such as pacing and energy conservation or pain management; accepting the need for and adjusting to use of assistive devices (including bilevel positive airway pressure); addressing anxiety about aging with a disability; developing plans for dealing with life transitions, such as retirement and role loss; assistance in explaining PPS and the polio experience to family members and significant others and improving communication around these issues; and processing grief around changed identity. Those patients with trauma-related issues report benefitting from the ability to integrate polio into trauma-informed treatment. Some patients have noted that because there is so little that can be done medically to ameliorate the condition, psychotherapy has been the most useful treatment they received. Others report that addressing the energy drain of unresolved psychological issues provides some improvement for their post–polio-related fatigue.

Directly and indirectly, patients have provided a wealth of information about the importance of a mental health–informed perspective in medical settings. Almost all endorse feeling heard and understood by their providers as an important element of their medical care, enabling them to raise sensitive topics they report that they otherwise would have avoided and creating corrective emotional experiences for past medical trauma. A positive relationship with a trusted physician or therapist often is reported as the reason for acceptance of the restrictions imposed by PPS, willingness to try assistive devices, and following-up on referrals, especially to mental health providers.

DISCUSSION

In an ideal world, there would be no stigma attached to seeing a mental health professional. Yearly wellness consultations with a mental health provider would be as routine as seeing an optometrist or dentist, with brief interventions prescribed as needed in order to address issues early. Unfortunately, even polio survivors who meet diagnostic criteria for major mental illness often go untreated. Medical providers may be reluctant to make referrals due to lack of knowledge of appropriate resources, skepticism about the efficacy of psychotherapy, or concern that patients will reject such referrals.

Finding appropriate referrals remains challenging. Although disability is the largest minority in the United States[27] and the only one anyone is eligible to join at any moment, there is a dearth of mental health professionals trained to work with people with disabilities, including polio. Many patients report having seen mental health professionals who minimized or ignored the effects of their polio experiences on their current functioning, failing to address significant issues around identity, body image, attachment, and medical trauma. The work they were able to do with these psychotherapists often was helpful and provided some relief. Once these individuals were given permission to bring their polio experiences into treatment, however, their conditions improved markedly.

In an ideal world, every polio clinic would include a mental health professional who routinely would see all new and returning patients (and, as desired and needed, their significant others). This person would provide consultation and training to the rehabilitation team. The resulting awareness of the psychological issues faced by polio survivors across the life span would inform all treatment provided by team members, each of whom would be comfortable utilizing this knowledge in discipline-appropriate ways. Referrals for longer-term services would be made to trusted psychotherapists both within and outside of the clinic, readily accepted by patients because of the confidence placed in these providers by the referring person and the clear explanation of the benefits of engaging in psychological treatment.

At least in the immediate future, this utopian vision is unlikely to become reality. Financial, institutional, space, and time constraints; lack of appropriately trained providers; and continued issues around destigmatizing mental health and educating all concerned about its place in the treatment of disability and chronic illness remain barriers to its fulfillment. Rehabilitation teams, however, can and should strive to create a culture of mental health, providing psychologically informed interventions appropriate to their roles and reaching out to appropriate mental health providers in the community for collaboration and training.

FUTURE DIRECTIONS

The COVID-19 pandemic has shown that telehealth is a viable option for treatment. Provided that the expansions Medicare and other insurers have permitted are maintained into the future and are coupled with changes in laws restricting interstate practice, polio survivors could benefit from being able to consult with specialists (including mental health professionals) from outside their immediate geographic area. Polio clinics likewise could benefit from the ability to virtually add a mental health professional to their staff, opening the potential for interprofessional collaboration and training over greater distances.

There is a need for more clinicians to be trained to work with polio survivors. As of 2006, it was conservatively estimated that there were 426,000 polio survivors in the United States.[28] According to Silver,[29] they constitute the second largest group of people with disabilities in the United States, with stroke being first. Because many who had polio as young children do not remember having had polio and were never told they had polio and because many who thought they had nonparalytic polio have gone on to develop PPS, this is thought to be an underestimate. Although a majority of polio survivors are over age 65, PPS does not shorten the life span. They, along with substantial numbers of younger polio survivors, including those born in the United States who had polio in the period 1955 to 1962 when yearly cases still numbered in the thousands, individuals born outside the United States in areas where polio remained endemic, and those whose polio was vaccine-induced, will need services for the foreseeable future. Reaching out to current practitioners in rehabilitation psychology, psychological trauma, and/or geropsychology to let them know that polio survivors still are here as well as providing polio-informed training experiences for the next generation would fill the need.

SUMMARY

When polio survivors' mental health issues are addressed by both medical and mental health providers, treatment outcomes improve. They report improved functioning and life satisfaction and are far more likely to comply with treatment. Unfortunately, more than 70 years after Morton Seidenfeld first attempted to raise awareness of their importance, these needs often are left unaddressed. It is my hope that this article inspires providers to try to change this and make his vision for integrated whole-person care a reality.

CLINICS CARE POINTS

- A polio-informed mental health consultation should be part of the full polio clinic evaluation, with treatment and/or referrals available as needed and desired.

- A polio-informed mental health provider needs a working knowledge of the physical and social issues related to polio, PPS, and disability in general. Given the prevalence of medical trauma in this population, training in psychological trauma is essential.

- Just as mental health professionals working with polio survivors need a discipline-appropriate working knowledge of their medical issues, physicians and therapists need a discipline-appropriate working knowledge of their psychological issues.

- Suffering caused by PPS may not be proportionate to the "objective" level of change or debility. "Passers" may have significantly more distress about smaller changes, whereas "identifiers" may be less concerned about identity issues related to changed disability status than "passers" or "minimizers" but more apprehensive about the implications of losing function.

- Many polio survivors have experienced trauma, including in medical settings. Providers should be alert to signs that that this may be the case, indicate openness to hearing whatever the patient wants to share, and provide empathy and appropriate referrals as needed.

DISCLOSURE

The author has nothing to disclose.

REFERENCES

1. Wilson DJ. Psychological trauma and its treatment in the polio epidemics. Bull Hist Med 2008;82(4):848–77.
2. Kaplan M. Psychology held major aid in polio. New York Times 1947.

3. Gallagher H. Blackbird fly away: disabled in an able-bodied world. Florida: Van-damere Press; 1998.
4. Kriegel L. Falling into life: essays. New York: North Point Press; 1991.
5. Davis F. Passage through crisis: polio victims and their families. Indianapolis (IN): Bobbs-Merrill; 1963.
6. Hubbard R. The psychologist working with crippled children. Ment Hyg 1944;28: 397–407.
7. Bibring G. Psychiatry and medical practice in a general hospital. N Engl J Med 1956;254:366–72.
8. Cohen E. A medical social worker's approach to the problem of poliomyelitis. Am J Public Health 1948;38:1092–6.
9. Meyer E. Psychological considerations in a group of children with poliomyelitis. J Pediatr 1944;31:34–48.
10. Finger A. Elegy for a disease: a personal and cultural history of polio. New York: St. Martin's Press; 2006.
11. Bruno RL, Frick NM. The psychology of polio as prelude to post-polio sequelae: Behavior modification and psychotherapy. Orthopedics 1991;14(11):1185–93.
12. Hammerlund SJ, Lexell J, Brogardh C. Perceived consequences of ageing with late effects of polio and strategies for managing daily life: A qualitative study. BMC Geriatr 2017;17:179.
13. Conrady LJ, Wish JR, Agre JC, et al. Psychologic characteristics of polio survi-vors: A preliminary report. Arch Phys Med Rehabil 1989;70:458–63.
14. Westbrook M, McIlwain D: Living with the late effects of disability: A five year follow-up survey of coping among post-polio survivors. Aust Occup Ther J 1996;43, 60-71.
15. Duncan A, Batliwalla Z. Growing older with post-polio syndrome: Social and qual-ity of life implications. SAGE Open Med 2018;6:1–7.
16. Kalpakjian CZ, Roller S, Tate DG. Psychological well-being of polio survivors. In: Silver JK, Gawne AC, editors. Postpolio syndrome. Philadelphia: Hanley and Bel-fus; 2004. p. 287–306.
17. Wilson DJ. Living with polio: the epidemic and its survivors. Chicago: University of Chicago Press; 2005.
18. Maynard F, Roller A. Recognizing typical coping styles of polio survivors can improve re-rehabilitation: A commentary. Am J Phys Med Rehabil 1991;70:70–2.
19. Halstead LS, Rossi CD. New problems in old polio patients: Results of a survey of 539 polio survivors. Orthopedics 1985;8(7):845–50.
20. Frick NM: Post-polio sequelae and the consequences of a second disability. Or-thopedics 1985; 8:7, 851-853.
21. Bakker M, Schipper K, Koopman FS, et al. Experiences and perspectives of pa-tients with post-polio syndrome and therapists with exercise and cognitive behav-ioral therapy. BMC Neurol 2016;16:23.
22. Wiley EAM: Aging with a long-term disability: Voices unheard. Phys Occup Ther Geriatr 2004;21:3, 33-47.
23. Opsvig AL. Ghosts of the past: polio survivors confront post-polio syndrome. Smith College, Northampton MA: Master's Thesis; 2011.
24. Bieniek LL, Kennedy K. Improving quality of life: Healing polio memories. Polio Netw News 2002;18(1):1–6.
25. Bieniek LL, Kennedy K. A guide for exploring polio memories. Polio Netw News 2002;18(3):3–6.
26. Bieniek LL, Kennedy K. Pursuing therapeutic resources to improve your health. Polio Netw News 2002;18(4):3–6.

27. Olkin R. What psychotherapists should know about disability. New York: Guilford; 1999.
28. Pierini D, Stuifbergen A. Psychological resilience and depressive symptoms in older adults diagnosed with post-polio syndrome. Rehabil Nurs 2010;35(4): 167–75.
29. Silver J. Talk at the 50th Anniversary of the Salk vaccine. Boston, MA: Children's Hospital; 2005.

Palliative Care for Polio and Postpolio Syndrome

John Y. Rhee, MD, MPH[a,b], Kate Brizzi, MD[a,c,d],*

KEYWORDS

- Palliative care • Polio • Symptom management • Advance care planning
- Caregiver support

KEY POINTS

- Palliative care is an approach to care that focuses on improving patients' quality of life through management of physical symptoms, psychosocial and existential distress, and support to the patient and family.
- A variety of symptoms can occur in polio and postpolio syndrome, including pain and contractures, hypersialorrhea, dyspnea, constipation, depression and anxiety, and fatigue.
- Early conversations with patients about their goals and values can help provide a framework for future care preferences.
- Palliative care is a team-based approach; a palliative care approach can be practiced by a primary care provider, bringing in a palliative care specialist when intensive symptom management is needed.

INTRODUCTION

Palliative care, according to the World Health Organization, is "an approach that improves the quality of life of patients and their families facing the problems associated with life-threatening illness, through the prevention and relief of suffering by means of early identification and impeccable assessment and treatment of pain and other problems, physical, psychosocial and spiritual."[1] Palliative care incorporates not only medication management for symptom relief but also coordination of support systems for patients and their families as they cope with an illness that shortens life-expectancy. Palliative care is a team-based approach, and includes doctors, nurses, nurse practitioners, social workers, psychologists, therapists, nutritionists, and chaplains to provide holistic care to the patient and family.

[a] Wang Ambulatory Care Center, Suite 835, 15 Parkman Street, Boston, MA 02114, USA; [b] Department of Neurology, Massachusetts General Hospital, Brigham and Women's Hospital, Harvard Medical School, Boston, MA, USA; [c] Department of Neurology, Massachusetts General Hospital, Boston, MA, USA; [d] Department of Medicine, Division of Palliative Care, Massachusetts General Hospital, Boston, MA, USA
* Corresponding author. Wang Ambulatory Care Center, Suite 835, 15 Parkman Street, Boston, MA 02114.
E-mail address: kbrizzi@partners.org

Phys Med Rehabil Clin N Am 32 (2021) 569–579
https://doi.org/10.1016/j.pmr.2021.02.008
1047-9651/21/© 2021 Elsevier Inc. All rights reserved.

Neuropalliative care is an emerging subspecialty within neurology that focuses on the approach to patients and their families who have life-limiting neurologic illnesses.[2] There are aspects of neuropalliative care that may be unique when compared with nonneurologic palliative care. For example, patients with serious neurologic illness may lose their ability to communicate early in their disease, as can be seen in motor neuron diseases such as amyotrophic lateral sclerosis or strokes affecting the language centers of the brain. Certain neurologic conditions, such as rapidly progressive dementias, may prevent patients from participating in medical decision-making early on, and many neurologic diseases are associated with behavioral changes that may create additional difficulties for caregivers and families. In addition, prognostication can be very variable and difficult to predict in neurologic diseases, and many diseases are characterized by uncertainty in relapses and recurrence.[3]

Furthermore, neurologic illnesses, more than other diseases, seem to have a large impact on the patient's sense of self, where patients "experience their disease as something intrinsic to their person, which clearly differs from patients with cancer who see 'the cancer' as something outside of themselves."[4]

Patients with neurologic illnesses often fall into 4 categories of disease trajectory: patients with rapid decline, patients with episodic decline, patients with prolonged decline, and patients presenting with acute crisis and uncertain recovery. Palliative care needs may vary among these different trajectories.

Poliomyelitis is caused by an enterovirus that damages the anterior horn motor cells of the spinal cord and brainstem, leading to cell death and disruption of motor units, with resultant muscle weakness or complete paralysis. Mortality of acute paralytic poliomyelitis can range from 2% to 5% among children and 15% to 30% in adults, with 25% to 75% mortality with bulbar involvement.[5] Palliative care for patients with poliomyelitis can fall into any of the first 3 categories of disease trajectory described earlier: patients with acute poliomyelitis with rapid decline, patients with biphasic form with further weakness after a short period of stability, or patients with postpolio syndrome or patients with previous paralytic poliomyelitis, which can show either episodic or prolonged decline over a period of many years.[6]

Palliative care is especially important in a life-limiting disease process that is chronic and progressive. Palliative care addresses patients holistically. In the case of patients with poliomyelitis, palliative care can help provide a framework approach to

1. Physical symptom management
2. Psychological aspects, including fears and concerns about the disease
3. Social aspects, such as coordinating resources for caregivers and families as well as supporting those close to the patient
4. Spiritual aspects such as reflecting on the meaning of life and fears of death and dying

Acute Paralytic Poliomyelitis and Postpolio Syndrome

Acute paralytic poliomyelitis consists of a meningitis phase, followed by spinal poliomyelitis with severe muscle pain and spasms, followed by weakness and fasciculations with lower greater than upper limb involvement. A purely bulbar form of poliomyelitis may also occur without limb weakness, particularly in children, whereas adults tend to have bulbar and spinal involvement. Although any cranial nerve may be involved, most commonly cranial nerves IX, X, XI, and XII are involved in the medulla, leading to dysphagia, dysphonia, and respiratory failure. High mortality rates usually occur from vasomotor disturbances and autonomic dysfunction such as hypertension, hypotension, and circulatory collapse as well as disturbances in micturition and gastroparesis. There is also a rare encephalitic form that manifests with agitation, confusion, stupor, and coma, which has a higher rate of autonomic dysfunction and mortality.[6]

Postpolio syndrome consists of new neurologic deficits after a prolonged period of neurologic stability, typically 15 years after the initial poliomyelitis infection, and symptoms include new persistent and progressive muscle weakness and atrophy, limb fatigability, myalgia, arthralgia, dysphagia, and generalized fatigue as well as cold intolerance and respiratory compromise.[7] Patients with postpolio syndrome are at increased risk for falls and may have a wide range of nonmotor symptoms such as sensory deficits and paresthesias as well as cognitive deficits such as word-finding difficulties, poor concentration, limited attention, memory impairment, and mood disturbances.[7] Fatigue can be exhibited through sleep disorders such as restless leg syndrome, sleep-related breathing disturbances, obstructive sleep apnea, excessive daytime somnolence, and periodic limb movement in sleep.[7] Orthopedic complications are very common and are due to prolonged abnormal stresses applied to joints due to muscle weakness, leading to progressive instability of joints, fractures, osteoporosis, osteoarthrosis, and scoliosis.[6] Because of the chronic nature of postpolio syndrome, respiratory insufficiency is also associated with progressive nocturnal hypoventilation due to chest wall deformity, progressive scoliosis, increased respiratory tract infections, and obstructive airway disease.[6]

Unfortunately, quantifying the rate of decline in postpolio syndrome is challenging, and no reliable functional predictors have been validated.[7]

DISCUSSION
Symptom Management in Poliomyelitis and Postpolio Syndrome

The symptoms discussed here may occur in both poliomyelitis as well as postpolio syndrome, with certain symptoms, such as fatigue and contractures, being more associated with postpolio syndrome and the acuity and severity of symptoms dependent on the phase of the disease. Therefore, any of the following can be applied to symptom management for the patient with either acute poliomyelitis or postpolio syndrome.

Hypersialorrhea
In patients with bulbar involvement, hypersialorrhea may put patients at risk for further respiratory distress as well as development of aspiration pneumonias, and symptoms of excess saliva may be uncomfortable and embarrassing for the patient.

Although there are no clinical trials testing the efficacy of one type of medication over another, oral medications are used as first-line therapy. Amitriptyline at low doses with its anticholinergic effects, can decrease excess secretions. The benefit of using amitriptyline is that it also can be used for (although at higher doses) anxiety/depression, pseudobulbar effect, insomnia, and chronic pain, although undesirable side effects include constipation and, in certain subgroups, an increased risk of delirium.[8] Other options include atropine drops 0.5% to 1% three or four times a day or glycopyrrolate solution 1 mg three times a day. For glycopyrrolate, the pill has variable absorption, and therefore, the solution is preferred over the tablet form. Transdermal hyoscine (scopolamine), 1.5 mg, exchanged every 3 days, can also be used, but it has side effects of confusion and loss of bladder control and may not be sufficient in controlling buccal secretions.[8]

When first-line oral medications are insufficient, botulinum toxin injections into the parotid and/or submandibular glands can help with controlling secretions, as well as radiation therapy to the glands, although short-term reversible side effects of thrush, pain, mouth sores, loss of taste, and worsening of dysphagia or dysarthria sometimes limit these interventions.[8]

Pain and contractures

Research shows that poliomyelitis survivors, especially those with more pain and fatigue symptoms, have poorer health-related quality of life.[9]

In the stage of acute infection, patients usually have severe headache associated with severe pain of the lower back accompanied by hyperesthesias of the skin, which may or may not be painful.[10] About 1 week later, after fevers have subsided, the headaches and hyperesthesias often improve, and patients are often left with low back pain and severe muscular pain that is worse with movement, pressure, and stretching. This pain, which can be severe, is often reported by patients when discussing poliomyelitis-associated pain.[10]

Headache can be managed with supportive acetaminophen or nonsteroidal antiinflammatory drugs (NSAIDs), with caution on frequency of dosing due to the possibility of developing rebound headache from medication overuse.

For pain associated with poliomyelitis, mechanisms that target vasodilation can often aid in some pain relief, including heat packs, neostigmine, as well as sympathetic blocks.[10] Preventive stretching is also important to prevent contractures, and NSAIDs and aspirin given before stretching can be given to assist in pain control. Involvement of physical and occupational therapy is important in helping to prevent contractures with stretching exercises.

Mobility aids are important to consider, to allow patients to maintain as much independence as possible, as well as to continue to maintain social relationships. Braces can support weakened muscles and joints (see Claudia A. Wheeler's article, "Bracing: Upper and Lower Limb Orthoses," in this issue), and walking sticks/trekking poles, electric scooters, or wheelchairs can aid in preserving mobility, especially for patients with postpolio syndrome.

Dyspnea and respiratory symptoms

Respiratory symptom management consists of airway management, management of secretions, control of dyspnea, and ventilator support. Most symptom management evidence is derived from work with patients with amyotrophic lateral sclerosis with lower motor neuron disease complications.

It is important that, within the interdisciplinary team, the patient is followed by a speech and language pathologist because uncoordinated swallowing, pooling of secretions, and vocal cord dysfunction can all contribute to the sensation of choking and breathlessness.[11] An effective cough is important in managing airway secretions. Patients can be taught assisted cough techniques, such as cough with abdominal thrust, usually with the help of a caregiver or through the help of mechanical cough devices.[11]

Secretions can become thickened in the setting of dehydration, which may often happen in patients who concurrently exhibit dysphagia and therefore may have decreased PO intake of thin liquids. Solutions for adequate hydration, either through percutaneous endoscopic gastrostomy (PEG) tube or scheduled fluids by mouth, can help prevent dehydration. In the more invasive realm, pharmacologic agents that can break up secretions such as acetylcysteine, 200 to 400 mg, three times a day or beta-receptor antagonists such as metoprolol or propranolol in a saline nebulizer with ipratropium or theophylline can assist in mobilization in conjunction with cough-assist techniques.[11] In relation to theophylline use, animal studies have noted increased diaphragmatic contractility, which may portend some benefit for airway clearance.[12–14] Portable suction devices can also help with secretions as well as humidification.

Judicious morphine in the setting of breathlessness is also an important tool. Benzodiazepines can also be helpful for tachypnea in the setting of anxiety. Studies in patients with amyotrophic lateral sclerosis have shown that the worry that morphine may worsen or precipitate respiratory failure is likely overemphasized, and morphine in doses ranging from 2 to 20 mg showed improvements in tachypnea without increases in carbon dioxide levels and with increases in oxygen levels.[15] The sensation of dyspnea can also be decreased with blowing cold air into the face with a small fan.

Noninvasive positive-pressure ventilation (NPPV) can improve symptoms of breathlessness, sleep, and cognitive function. NPPV can be delivered by nasal or a full-face mask.[11] Nasal discomfort is a common discomfort for patients starting on NPPV. Anticholinergic nasal spray can be used to treat rhinorrhea and nasal congestion relieved through a humidifier. Abdominal bloating from excessive air swallowing can be treated with promotility agents such as metoclopramide.

Constipation
Patients with poliomyelitis and postpolio syndrome can experience severe constipation, which is likely multifactorial in nature. Decreased mobility, changes in hydration and oral intake, medications, and autonomic dysfunction can all play a role in increasing constipation. A step-up strategy for treatment of constipation that is often used in patients with constipation, in general, can be applied to this patient population.

The overall goal is to try to maintain a daily, scheduled bowel movement, preferably around the same time daily as well as maintaining a high fiber diet with sufficient fluids. Psyllium and methylcellulose can be added to the diet to increase fiber, although, of note, without sufficient fluids, a diet high in fiber will not necessarily improve bowel movements. Daily bowel movements are important in order to create a habit and schedule for bowel movements as well as to prevent bowel distention from accumulation of stool, which further decreases the ability of the bowels for effective peristalses to evacuate the stool.

The next step, if needed, is to schedule laxatives. Osmotic (polyethylene glycol, lactulose) and stimulant laxative (senna tablets) agents can be added sequentially in order to ensure daily bowel movements, with uptitration, as needed. Suppositories (bisacodyl or glycerin) can also be used, as needed, to ensure daily bowel movements, and peeled off when a regular bowel movement schedule is achieved. Recent studies have found docusate sodium to be ineffective[16] and may not help with softening stools, instead, adding to pill burden.[17]

If a patient has not had a bowel movement for 3 or more days, disimpaction may be necessary to allow for decreased bowel distension as well as to clear out hard, impacted stool.

Anxiety/depression
Patients with postpolio syndrome, when compared with matched healthy controls as well as mobility-limited controls, still seem to have a greater burden of anxiety.[9] However, in general, patients with serious illnesses such as poliomyelitis should not be assumed to develop an anxiety or depressive disorder, although they may experience heightened levels of fears or worries about their future. For many patients, a period of adjustment may be a natural process of coping with illness. However, when symptoms become debilitating pharmacotherapy may be necessary to prevent the extremes of anxiety or depression, that is, the desire to shorten life in order to escape from these symptoms. Untreated anxiety can result in more fatigue, pain, dyspnea, and an overall sense of well-being, and depression can limit the ability of a patient to fully participate in end-of-life care.[18]

In the case of adjustment to disease, patients may benefit from a wide range of support to help them through the coping process. Maintaining a strong social network is important as well as a trusting relationship between the patient and health care team. An assessment of lifestyle factors, including sleep hygiene, caffeine intake, or other drug use, is a first-line measure.

Where pharmacotherapy becomes necessary, benzodiazepines may be used to treat acute attacks of anxiety, whereas selective serotonin reuptake inhibitors can be used to treat chronic anxiety or depression. For benzodiazepines, the lowest dose should always be chosen, with uptitration, as needed. Medications such as tricyclic antidepressants, although with many side effects, can be considered for their multipurpose effects, including management of secretions, depression, and/or assistance with sleep.

Fatigue and sleep disturbances

Fatigue can be debilitating for patients, especially for those with postpolio syndrome. Reversible causes should be ruled out first as well as implementation of lifestyle changes before progression to pharmacotherapy. As mentioned earlier, poliomyelitis survivors, especially those with more pain and fatigue symptoms, have poorer health-related quality of life.[9] In the palliative care setting, it is important to distinguish fatigue from weakness, depression, drowsiness, existential distress, or psychomotor slowing. Fatigue is defined as "a subjective state characterized by feelings of tiredness and a perception of decreased capacity for physical or mental work."[19]

Treatment can be based on preventative and reversible causes of fatigue. If a patient is anemic, depending on the cause of anemia, they may be treated with supplementation as well as consideration of transfusion for symptomatic improvement. Although there have been no research on improvement in fatigue with higher transfusion goals in patients with postpolio syndrome, in patients with advanced cancer, a goal of 8 g/dL improved symptoms of fatigue in a subset of patients.[20]

Nonpharmacologic interventions include scheduled exercise, maintaining good sleep hygiene with consistent sleep-wake cycles, including phototherapy, where necessary, to aid in keeping awake during the day, and cognitive behavioral therapy. There is no robust evidence to suggest pharmacologic interventions. Most of the literature is dedicated to fatigue in patients with cancer, which may not be directly applicable to patients with postpolio syndrome. Low doses of dexamethasone can be trialed, as well as psychostimulants such as modafinil or methylphenidate for fatigue that may be related to opioids.

Sleep disorders are common not just in poliomyelitis or postpolio syndrome but in patients with other neuromuscular disorders as well.[21] Similarly to fatigue, reversible causes should first be identified, such as discomfort or pain, switching of sleep-wake cycles or long naps during the day, sleep hygiene including reducing caffeine intake or screen time, and ensuring a cool, quiet, and dark environment at nighttime.

Pharmacologic interventions can be trialed, especially where there may be a dual benefit. For example, mirtazapine can be used at bedtime, with the additional benefit of treatment of depression as well as weight gain. Melatonin and melatonin-receptor agonists such as ramelteon have few side effects, given melatonin is also naturally produced by the body, and can be used before bedtime. In general, avoiding anticholinergics may assist in preventing worsening of delirium, although medications such as amitriptyline can also be used for depression and secretions in addition to sleep, when given at bedtime.

> **Box 1**
> **Triggers for serious illness conversations in addition to routine check-ins[23]**
>
> 1. A new diagnosis
> 2. A change in therapeutic plan
> 3. A major change in management
> 4. A transfer to another institution
> 5. Continued patient discomfort and/or difficulties managing symptoms
> 6. If the patient or family asks to discuss this topic
> 7. Major decrease in functional capacity
> 8. Frequent hospitalization
>
> *Data from* Creutzfeldt CJ, Robinson MT, Holloway RG. Neurologists as primary palliative care providers: Communication and practice approaches. *Neurol Clin Pract.* 2016;6(1):40-48.

Cognitive or behavioral changes and delirium

Delirium is common in the acute phase of poliomyelitis with subsequent return to baseline over a 2-week period.[19] Symptoms of delirium can include acute fluctuations in attention, frank delusions, and visual hallucinations. Rarely, patients may remember these experiences.[22]

As is the case in delirium in other neurologic conditions, patients should first be assessed for any underlying cause of the delirium. Assessment should include evaluation for delirium secondary to certain sedating or prodopaminergic or anticholinergic medications, infection, withdrawal, and pain. Frequent orientation of the patient, with the help of people the patient is familiar with, such as family members, using clear and concise communication, keeping the room light during the day and dark at night, reducing noise, and limiting staff changes, can all help a patient in reducing the risk of or severity of delirium.[15] If nonpharmacological methods are ineffective, pharmacologic interventions can be attempted. The first-line pharmacologic treatment of delirium is neuroleptics, such as haloperidol or atypical antipsychotics such as olanzapine, risperidone, quetiapine, and aripiprazole, which tend to have fewer extrapyramidal side effects when compared with haloperidol.

Goals of Care and Serious Illness Discussions

Goals of care

There are also some natural points along the disease process where trigger situations invite the patient, family, and provider to reflect again on goals of care in addition to routine check-ins (**Box 1**).

In general, a 6-step protocol[24] is advised for initiating a goals-of-care conversation.

1. Prepare and establish an appropriate setting for the discussion.
2. Ask the patient and family what they understand.
3. Find out what they expect will happen.
4. Discuss overall goals and specific options.
5. Respond to emotions.
6. Establish and implement the plan.

Throughout these steps, clinicians should be aware of the balance of listening versus speaking, being empathetic to emotions, and responding appropriately. There should be more listening, and where a clinician feels he/she is speaking too much, he/she should take a step back and allow the family or patient to speak.

To these steps discussed earlier, the authors also add a seventh, which include feedback at the end of a goals-of-care conversation. Ideally, a more experienced clinician will observe a clinician-in-training leading a goals-of-care conversation and provide feedback in order to continue the process of learning and improving communication skills.

One aspect of serious illness conversations is advanced directives. Advanced directives are an important way to preserve the wishes of the patient, while understanding the important caveat that patient's preferences can change over time and over the disease course. The most important role of the physician is to initiate discussions on advanced directives, both to better educate the patient and to encourage the patient to think of what he/she would like in certain scenarios and how they would like to be treated medically in those scenarios. Ideally, these discussions would be had with the patient and the health care proxy present, so that the proxy can accurately represent the patient's preferences, should the need arise.

In the discussion process, certain questions could help guide the decision-making process.

1. Would the patient want to stay at home in the case of an emergency or escalate care?
2. Code status: would the patient want to be made DNR (do not resuscitate) or DNI (do not intubate) or both?
3. Gastrostomy and tracheostomy
4. Who would the patient want to be notified in the case of an emergency?
5. Health care proxy form

As emphasized earlier, these discussions should be recurrent and readdressed periodically; this also encourages the patient and family to readdress some of these topics over time after discussion with family and friends. Furthermore, goals-of-care should not be seen as a conversation in a single point in time, but rather, should be seen as a larger process that evolves over a period of time. Here, it is important to be aware of one's personal biases as well as institutional biases, which may include cultural biases as well as, for example, the bias in medicine where there is a desire to gather information quickly and efficiently, whereas a process may require more time and prolonged discussion through a period that may include multiple intermediary steps from denial to acceptance.

Transitions in care: nutrition, tracheostomy, and hospice

The key to transitions is early conversations with patients about their wishes and desires if their disease process were to progress. It is important to focus on the patient as a person and his/her values, seeking to better understand a patient's understanding, hopes, worries, and values to help provide a framework for future decision-making, rather than focusing on a specific decision.[25]

For some patients, discussions may clearly indicate that a surgical procedure, even though minor, for a gastrostomy tube insertion or tracheostomy is not within their goals of care. However, a small proportion of patients can change their mind as the disease progresses, and therefore, readdressing these questions is of vital importance. Furthermore, gastrostomy tube placement and tracheostomy can be congruent to a patient's desires, even in a palliative care setting, and can even alleviate some distressing symptoms, with the understanding that palliative PEG and tracheostomy are not for curing the underlying disease process and/or may not prolong life but rather to provide symptom support within a patient's goals in the long run.[26,27]

A patient and/or patient's family may decide to switch over to a comfort-directed care, at which point a patient can be transitioned to hospice care if he/she has a life-expectancy of 6 months or less. In discussions with patients and their families about transitioning to hospice care, it is important to indicate to them that, at no point in their decision-making process is a decision irreversible. This sometimes helps provide some mental comfort for patients and families when transitioning over to hospice care and can provide an intermediary step in that transition. Important themes to touch on include confirming code status as well as whether a patient would want to be brought into the hospital in the case of an emergency or whether they would want to stay at home with the aid of the hospice agency to provide comfort care.

Coping and Caregiver Support

Part of the palliative care team's role is to also ensure that caregivers of patients are supported. This results in better care for the patient as well as ensures the well-being of those closest to the patient in what can be a chronic disease process, such as postpolio. The health care provider can assist the caregiver, who is the primary care-taker of the patient, by engaging multiple family members in the care of the patient, trying to attain a good sleep-wake cycle to allow the caregiver to rest, and working with the interdisciplinary team for support in day programs, legal and financial issues related to the patient's care, and, where appropriate, psychological counseling for the caregiver as well as connecting the caregiver to support groups. Such precautions help prevent the caregiver from also becoming a patient and may help offload some of the difficulties the caregiver may experience in a chronic process such as postpolio syndrome, but can also apply to the acute setting in acute poliomyelitis, where additional emotional burden may have a toll on the patient's loved ones and support system.

Interprofessional Care

The palliative care approach can be used by many different types of providers, and ideally, high-quality palliative care is delivered by an interprofessional team. In the case of acute poliomyelitis as well as postpolio syndrome, optimal care requires input from the whole team. The patients' primary physician, whether that be a primary care physician, physiatrist, palliative care physician, or neurologist, plays an important palliative care role in assessing and treating symptoms, cultivating prognostic awareness, and encouraging early conversations about goals and values. Physical and occupational therapists assist with stretching and adjusting to limitations in the home and work settings. Speech and language pathologists monitor and advise on bulbar dysfunction and aspiration risk and provide valuable input on when feeding tubes need to be considered. Nutritionists can aid in assisting with preventing weight loss, which can arise from a variety of factors including fatigue, depression, aspiration risk, and difficulties coordinating swallowing. Chaplains play very important roles in providing assistance to patients who are experiencing existential distress. Research shows that existential distress at the end of life can be one of the most debilitating symptoms for patients who are dying, and so this role is of critical importance.[28] Psychologists and/or social workers can provide counseling and nonpharmacological interventions for patients having difficulties adjusting to their new limitations and/or with new diagnoses of depression or anxiety. Palliative nurses provide important support to patients and are able to best notice when patients are suffering from a wide range of symptoms. This team approach is important in a disease such as acute poliomyelitis, where the initial stages of the disease can be unpredictable, and loss of function can be very rapid, as well as in postpolio syndrome, where the chronic process of periods of deterioration and periods of stability can cause a lot of frustration for patients as well as fears and anxieties.

A palliative care approach is important in the care of patients with polio and postpolio syndrome and should be initiated early in the course of a patient's care. Early palliative care has been shown to improve mood and quality of life and in certain cases, paradoxically, longer survival.[29] Early palliative care involvement for patients suffering from acute poliomyelitis and referral when patients are diagnosed with postpolio syndrome may help provide more comprehensive care to the patient and allow for a better quality of life.

CLINICS CARE POINTS

- Palliative care is applicable at any stage of illness, even at the time of diagnosis.

- Sialorrhea can be treated with anticholinergic medications, although providers should monitor for side effects such as dry mouth, constipation, and confusion. Botox can be helpful for refractory cases.

- Dyspnea unresponsive to nonmedication approaches can be treated with low-dose opioids.

- Triggers for serious illness conversations include difficulty with managing symptoms, changes in functional capacity, frequent hospitalizations, or a change in the therapeutic plan.

DISCLOSURE

The authors have nothing to disclose.

REFERENCES

1. World Health Organization. Definition of Palliative Care. Available at: https://www. who.int/health-topics/palliative-care. Accessed August 2020.
2. Creutzfeldt CJ, Kluger B, Kelly AG, et al. Neuropalliative care: Priorities to move the field forward. Neurology 2018;91(5):217–26.
3. Brizzi K, Creutzfeldt CJ. Neuropalliative care: a practical guide for the neurologist. Semin Neurol 2018;38(5):569–75.
4. Boersma I, Miyasaki J, Kutner J, et al. Palliative care and neurology: time for a paradigm shift. Neurology 2014;83(6):561–7.
5. Center for Disease Control. Poliomyelitis. 2020. Available at: https://www.cdc.gov/vaccines/pubs/pinkbook/polio. Accessed April 2021.
6. Kidd D, Williams AJ, Howard RS. Poliomyelitis. Postgrad Med J 1996;72(853): 641–7.
7. Li Hi Shing S, Chipika RH, Finegan E, et al. Post-polio syndrome: more than just a lower motor neuron disease. Front Neurol 2019;10:773.
8. Karam CY, Paganoni S, Joyce N, et al. Palliative care issues in amyotrophic lateral sclerosis: an evidenced-based review. Am J Hosp Palliat Care 2016;33(1):84–92.
9. Yang EJ, Lee SY, Kim K, et al. Factors associated with reduced quality of life in polio survivors in Korea. PLoS One 2015;10(6):e0130448.
10. Guyton AC, Reeder RC. Pain and contracture in poliomyelitis. Arch Neurol Psychiatry 1950;63(6):954–63.
11. Gelinas D. Respiratory complications. Palliative care in amyotrophic lateral sclerosis: from diagnosis to bereavement. 3rd edition. Oxford Scholarship Online; 2014.

12. Aubier M, DeTroyer A, Sampson M, et al. Aminophylline improves diaphragmatic contractility. N Engl J Med 1981;305:249–52.
13. Murciano D, Aubier M, Lecocguic Y, et al. Effects of theophylline on diaphragmatic strength and fatigue in patients with chronic obstructive pulmonary disease. N Engl J Med 1984;311:349–53.
14. Foxworth JW, Reisz GR, Knudson SM, et al. Theophylline and diaphragmatic contractility: investigation of a dose response relationship. Am Rev Respir Dis 1988;138:1532–4.
15. Clemens KE, Klaschik E. Morphine in the management of dyspnoea in ALS. A pilot study. Eur J Neurol 2008;15(5):445–50.
16. Canadian Agency for Drugs and Technologies in Health. Dioctyl sulfosuccinate or docusate (calcium or sodium) for the prevention or management of constipation: a review of the clinical effectiveness. Online Report. 2014.
17. Ramkumar D, Rao SS. Efficacy and safety of traditional medical therapies for chronic constipation: systematic review. Am J Gastroenterol 2005;100(4):936–71.
18. Bush SL, Gagnon B, Lawlor PG. Delirium. Palliative Medicine: a case-based manual. Oxford Scholarship Online; 2012.
19. Stone P, Richards M, Hardy J. Fatigue in patients with cancer. Eur J Cancer 1998; 34(11):1670–6.
20. Preston NJ, Hurlow A, Brine J, et al. Blood transfusions for anaemia in patients with advanced cancer. Cochrane Database Syst Rev 2012;(2):CD009007.
21. Araujo MA, Silva TM, Moreira GA, et al. Sleep disorders frequency in post-polio syndrome patients caused by periodic limb movements. Arq Neuropsiquiatr 2010;68(1):35–8.
22. Holland JC, Coles MR. Neuropsychiatric aspects of acute poliomyelitis. Am J Psychiatry 1957;114(1):54–63.
23. Creutzfeldt CJ, Robinson MT, Holloway RG. Neurologists as primary palliative care providers: Communication and practice approaches. Neurol Clin Pract 2016;6(1):40–8.
24. Vollrath AM, von Gunten CF. Chapter 4 - Negotiating Goals of Care: Changing Goals Along the Trajectory of Illness. In: Emanuel LL, Librach SL, editors. Palliative care. 2nd edition. W.B. Saunders; 2011. p. 56–68.
25. Paladino J, Bernacki R, Neville BA, et al. Evaluating an intervention to improve communication between oncology clinicians and patients with life-limiting cancer: a cluster randomized clinical trial of the serious illness care program. JAMA Oncol 2019;5(6):801–9.
26. Goldberg LS, Altman KW. The role of gastrostomy tube placement in advanced dementia with dysphagia: a critical review. Clin Interv Aging 2014;9:1733–9.
27. Chan T, Devaiah AK. Tracheostomy in palliative care. Otolaryngol Clin North Am 2009;42(1):133–41, x.
28. Boston P, Bruce A, Schreiber R. Existential suffering in the palliative care setting: an integrated literature review. J Pain Symptom Manage 2011;41(3):604–18.
29. Temel JS, Greer JA, Muzikansky A, et al. Early palliative care for patients with metastatic non-small-cell lung cancer. N Engl J Med 2010;363(8):733–42.

Health Care Delivery, Patient Resources, and Community Reintegration

Jenna Raheb, PT, DPT, PCS[a,b,c,*]

KEYWORDS

- Multidisciplinary • Patient centered • Adaptive equipment • Accessibility
- Adaptive sports • Caregiving

KEY POINTS

- Use of multidisciplinary clinics should be considered when working with medically complex patients. Health care should be provided in a patient-centered and family-centered manner.
- Wheeled mobility and adaptive equipment should be considered for patients when it can allow increased independence, health benefits, and/or reduced caregiver burden.
- The home, work, and community environments can be adapted to improve accessibility for people with disabilities.
- Physical activity and adaptive sports should be encouraged and discussed with patients with disabilities. Guidelines regarding safety as it pertains to the patient and the diagnosis should be reviewed with the patient and family.
- The health and well-being of caregivers needs to be considered and looked after.

HEALTH CARE DELIVERY FOR MEDICALLY COMPLEX PATIENTS
Multidisciplinary Teams

Patients with complex medical diagnoses benefit from being followed by multidisciplinary clinics. Multidisciplinary clinics are composed of a variety of different health care professionals that specialize in the diagnosis of the patient population seen by that clinic. These clinicians can evaluate the patients at a low frequency (ie, monthly, yearly, and so forth). The clinicians in a multidisciplinary clinic can provide care and referrals while monitoring patients in different stages of the disease process, and they evaluate the patients from their own clinical perspectives. For example, children with cerebral palsy (CP) should be followed by a multidisciplinary CP clinic regularly. During their clinic visits, they should have consultations with clinicians such as physical medicine and rehabilitation physicians, orthopedic physicians, nurses, orthotists,

[a] Raheb Physical Therapy; [b] Boston University; [c] Spaulding Rehabilitation Hospital
* Corresponding author.
E-mail address: jraheb@bu.edu

Phys Med Rehabil Clin N Am 32 (2021) 581–589
https://doi.org/10.1016/j.pmr.2021.02.009
1047-9651/21/© 2021 Elsevier Inc. All rights reserved.

physical therapists, occupational therapists, and speech therapists, all of whom specialize in working with patients with CP. At these clinics, other professionals, such as case managers and social workers, can meet with families to provide support in various ways. As the children with CP age, clinicians guide the families with recommendations such as surgeries; muscle tone management; medication; bracing and equipment needs; and referrals to physical, occupational, and speech therapy. They can also monitor for changes in joint range of motion and hip development, common areas of impairment in this population.

The multidisciplinary clinic model is one that has been used for many years. Research shows that this model provides improved patient outcomes[1,2] and reductions in patient mortality.[1,3] Research also shows that this model is cost-effective[3] and can even reduce health care costs.[2]

Interdisciplinary Teams

In the multidisciplinary approach described earlier, clinicians evaluate and treat patients from their own perspectives. There is communication among team members, but not always. In the interdisciplinary team model, clinicians from different disciplines work together when evaluating and treating patients. There is regular communication and collaboration among the team members. They work together toward common goals to evaluate and treat patients. This type of care is common in settings such as inpatient rehabilitation. Research shows that this model allows improved patient outcomes and can reduce health care costs.[4]

Because referrals are made to other health care professionals, such as outpatient speech therapists, outpatient occupational and physical therapists, and orthotists, there should be communication and collaboration among team members to provide the best care. Patients are commonly seen by clinicians that work for separate companies or hospitals, which can make communication between health care professionals difficult. However, clinicians across settings should have some form of communication as they are caring for their patients.

Frequency of Outpatient Therapy Services

Patients with complex medical diagnoses often require outpatient therapies, such as occupational therapy and physical therapy, for many years. These therapists should consider the episodic care model when determining frequencies. Physicians should also educate families on this model of care when recommending these services. When providing episodic care, clinicians are providing a particular service for a specific problem for a particular period of time.[5] When determining the frequency of delivery, factors that are considered include, but are not limited to, the patient's ability to participate, the amount of clinical decision making required, the level of family support, and the potential for progression or regression. This frequency should be regularly evaluated and adjusted as appropriate.[6]

For example, an adult patient who has had a stroke with a resultant decline in function may require care in an acute care hospital followed by an inpatient rehabilitation hospital. In these settings and at this stage of recovery where rapid improvement occurs, the patient typically receives a high frequency of therapy services (ie, daily). When the patient is discharged from inpatient rehabilitation, the patient may require outpatient services if the patient is expected to continue to make progress. At this point, the expected rate of progress is slower, so the frequency may be reduced (ie, 1 to 3 times per week). When the patient's progress slows or when the patient is unable to attend as many sessions, the frequency may reduce further. When the patient plateaus or when skilled intervention is no longer required, the patient may be discharged. After discharge, the patient may return to outpatient services if there is a change in the patient's function or if other needs, such as for adaptive equipment, need to be met.

When a patient has a progressive disorder, maintenance therapy is often recommended to improve functional outcomes, provide education and training to the patient and family over the course of the progression of the disease, and sometimes slow the negative impacts of the disorder (eg, reduced range of motion). In this scenario, the frequency also depends on the expected risk and rate of regression if therapy services are not provided. The frequency of service also depends on how much therapy services are expected to affect the therapeutic goals listed earlier.

Family-centered and Patient-centered Care

It is well documented in the literature that patient outcomes are improved when patient-centered and family-centered care is provided. The patient's and caregivers' goals and concerns should always be considered. They provide insight and information that is vital to providing good health care. Not only does patient-centered and family-centered care provide for better patient care and outcomes, it also allows for improved patient and family satisfaction, more cost-effective care, improved staff satisfaction, and reduced medical errors.[7]

What is considered to be evidence based is not always what the patient and family wish to follow. It is important that the patient and family are educated on their options and what is medically recommended, but the clinician needs to work as a team with the patient and family to figure out what the best plan of care is for the patient and family and what is feasible for them. Clinicians often have to alter their recommendations to accommodate what the patient's and caregivers' needs and wishes are.

IMPROVING PATIENT INDEPENDENCE AND ACCESS
Wheeled Mobility

When a patient has difficulty with navigating the home and community environments using walking as the means of mobility, wheeled mobility should be considered. If the expectation is that the patient will only require wheeled mobility for a short period of time, options such as rental wheelchairs, transport chairs, or electric scooters should be considered. If the patient will require a wheelchair for long-term use, a custom wheelchair that is tailored to the patient and the patient's needs should be considered.

To initiate the process of obtaining a custom wheelchair, the patient should be referred to an outpatient physical therapist who specializes in wheelchairs or a wheelchair clinic. The physical therapist should work with a vendor and/or equipment companies to provide trials of different wheelchairs. To make sure patients obtain the proper wheelchair for their needs, they should trial different wheelchairs and educate themselves on different options and features. The physical therapist and vendor work with the patient and family to provide education on different types of wheelchairs, wheelchair features, and the process of obtaining equipment.

Any functional limitations that the patient has at home and within the community should be documented in physician notes. During the ordering process, physician documentation is required and needs to support the request for a wheelchair. When referring the patient to the physical therapist, the physician should communicate with the physical therapist what the physician's concerns are, any prognostic information, any precautions, any past and future surgeries, other past and future medical interventions, as well as any functional limitations that prompted the referral.

After completing wheelchair trials, the patient and family meet with the patient's physical therapist and a vendor. The vendor, and sometimes the physical therapist, are assistive technology professionals. The patient, family, physical therapist, and vendor work together to determine the most appropriate choice of wheelchair and create a specifications list, which includes all of the features and accessories that the wheelchair will have. The physical therapist then writes a letter of medical necessity. The vendor provides the physician with the letter of medical necessity, the specifications list, a prescription to be signed, and potentially some additional forms the physician needs to fill out. The vendor asks for supporting documentation from the physician. The vendor collects all documentation and submits a request for coverage to insurance. If insurance coverage for the wheelchair is denied by the insurance company, the patient, family, physical therapist, and vendor need to work together to figure out why it was denied and what can be done in order to get insurance approval. This process typically requires reaching out to the insurance company for more information. Sometimes this requires reaching out to the manufacturer of the wheelchair to seek support and guidance. Depending on the reason for denial, alterations can be made to the specifications list, letter of medical necessity, and/or other supporting documentation, and the request can then be resubmitted. If the patient is not seeking insurance coverage, the process of submitting for insurance approval can be skipped (Fig. 1).

The role of the physical therapist described earlier can be completed by an occupational therapist as well who specializes in wheelchairs. Input may also be sought from other clinicians as appropriate. If the patient is receiving inpatient care, has a new diagnosis and/or recent functional decline, and needs a custom wheelchair, this process can be initiated in the inpatient setting.

On receipt of the wheelchair, patient and caregiver training should be completed for proper use of the wheelchair.

When considering wheeled mobility, there are many options to consider depending on the needs of the patient. There are a variety of different manual wheelchairs and power wheelchairs. There are also power assist devices that can be added to assist the patient with propulsion of a manual wheelchair. As stated previously, there are also electric scooters and transport wheelchairs. Insurance companies typically have a limit as to how many wheelchairs they will cover (ie, 1 wheelchair every 5 years), so, when providing prognostic information and concerns to the physical therapist, this should be considered.

If clinicians, patients, or families are looking for educational resources to expand their knowledge base on wheelchairs, they can refer to the Rehabilitation Engineering and Assistive Technology Society of North America (RESNA) Web site, resna.org. There are a variety of resources on this Web site, including position papers and service provision guidelines.[8]

Adaptive Equipment

Adaptive equipment is another useful tool for patients. Adaptive equipment are devices that are used to assist with activities of daily living and mobility. They can reduce caregiver burden and provide health benefits. For example, adaptive shower chairs can allow patients who cannot stand in the shower safely to sit in the shower to bathe themselves. It also makes it easier for the caregiver to assist the patient. Patients who do not spend a sufficient amount of time standing often get adaptive standers. Standers allow the maintenance of or increase in bone mineral density, maintenance and/or improvement in joint range of motion, reduced spasticity in the lower extremity muscles, and improved mental function.[9] There are many types of simple, adaptive

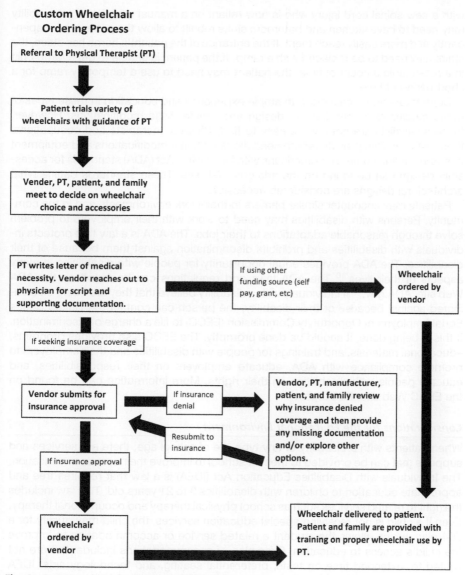

Custom Wheelchair Ordering Process

Referral to Physical Therapist (PT)

↓

Patient trials variety of wheelchairs with guidance of PT

↓

Vender, PT, patient, and family meet to decide on wheelchair choice and accessories

↓

PT writes letter of medical necessity. Vendor reaches out to physician for script and supporting documentation.

→ If using other funding source (self pay, grant, etc) → Wheelchair ordered by vendor

If seeking insurance coverage

↓

Vendor submits for insurance approval

→ If insurance denial → Vendor, PT, manufacturer, patient, and family review why insurance denied coverage and then provide any missing documentation and/or explore other options.

Resubmit to insurance

If insurance approval

↓

Wheelchair ordered by vendor

Wheelchair delivered to patient. Patient and family are provided with training on proper wheelchair use by PT.

Fig. 1. Custom wheelchair ordering process

equipment that are readily available in stores. There are also more custom and durable equipment that can be obtained in the same way that patients obtain a custom wheelchair (described earlier).

As with wheelchairs, patient and caregiver training should be completed for proper and safe use of equipment.

Home, Work, and Community Accessibility

Another way home access can be improved is through home modifications. This method is something that may need to occur with changing functional status and/or initiation of using a wheelchair or other adaptive equipment. For example, a patient with a new spinal cord injury who is now reliant on a manual wheelchair for mobility may need to have kitchen and bathroom sinks rebuilt to allow the patient to independently and more easily reach them. If the entrance of the patient's home has stairs, the stairs may need to be replaced with a ramp. If the patient is unable to get a ramp built in a reasonable amount of time, the patient may need to use a temporary ramp for a short period of time.

Contractors and architects with ample experience and education in these types of home modifications can help to design and create these modifications. However, these specialists are not always easy to find. Physical therapists and occupational therapists can also provide recommendations on home modifications and equipment needs within the home. The Americans with Disabilities Act (ADA) standards for accessible design can be found on the ada.gov Web site. These standards outline what architectural designs are considered accessible.

Patients may encounter similar barriers in their work environments and in the community. Persons with disabilities may need to work with their employers to problem solve through reasonable adaptations to their jobs. The ADA is a law that protects individuals with disabilities and prohibits discrimination against them because of their disabilities. The ADA provides equal opportunity for people with disabilities in many aspects of their lives.[10] The ADA laws and regulations can be found on the ADA Web site, ADA.gov.[11] If individuals with a disability believe that they are being discriminated against because of their disability, the person can contact the United States Equal Employment Opportunity Commission (EEOC) to file a charge of discrimination. If this is being done, it should be done promptly. The EEOC also provides programs, educational materials, and trainings for people with disabilities and their employers to promote compliance with ADA, educate employers on their responsibilities, and educate people with disabilities on their rights. More information can be found on the EEOC Web site, EEOC.gov.[12]

Considerations for the Educational Environment

When patients with a disability of any type are of school age, there are services and supports that can be provided to them at school to improve their access to education. The Individuals with Disabilities Education Act (IDEA) is a law that requires free and appropriate education to children with disabilities 3 to 21 years old. This law includes the right to related services such as school physical therapy and occupational therapy. Even if a child is not receiving special education services, the child may qualify for a 504 plan, which allows the student a related service or accommodation to improve the child's access to education. Examples of accommodations include, but are not limited to, extended time on tests, preferential seating, and technology aids. IDEA also incorporates assistance with transitions, including the transition from high school to the community.[13,14]

If a patient with a disability is attending a college or university, the patient should contact the office of disabilities of that school to discuss the patient's needs and find out what resources are available at the school.

PHYSICAL FITNESS AND ADAPTIVE SPORTS

Youth with physical and intellectual disabilities participate in less physical activity than their age-matched peers. Research also shows that children with disabilities participate in their preferred choice of physical activity less frequently and participate in fewer day-to-day physical recreation activities such as walking and cycling.[15]

There are a variety of barriers to participation in physical activity and adaptive sports in this population, such as limited financial resources, transportation barriers, and lack of resources in the areas the patients live. Clinicians should encourage their patients to participate in physical activity and help to connect them with the appropriate resources and clinicians to guide them.[16] It is well supported in the research that patients with disabilities should participate in regular physical activity. Physical activity has both physical and psychological benefits and can improve patients' quality of life.[16,17]

When guiding patients with a disability through physical activity recommendations, general health and safety concerns should be discussed, such as heat safety, the importance of proper hydration, and the importance of injury prevention programs and strategies. Diagnosis-specific concerns should be addressed. For example, patients with spinal cord injuries should be educated on autonomic dysreflexia, sensory impairments, skin health, low bone mineral density, neurogenic bladder and bowel, and thermoregulation. Patients with amputations should be educated on skin health and the importance of properly fitting and maintained prosthetic devices.[16]

PATIENT SUPPORT SYSTEMS
Peer Mentors and Mentees

People with disabilities may benefit from being connected with someone who has the same or a similar disability. This peer mentor can provide them emotional support, share personal experiences, and share resources. Being placed in the role of the peer mentor can also be a helpful and rewarding experience. With proper permissions from patients and abiding by patient privacy laws, clinicians can help to connect patients and families with each other. Clinicians should be aware of support groups and mentor programs in their areas. Clinicians can also start and coordinate support groups for their patient populations.

Caring for the Caregivers

People both with and without disabilities are living longer. With the increase in the elderly and disabled population, the need for caregiving has increased. According to the Centers for Disease Control and Prevention (CDC), between 2000 and 2030 the population of people aged 65 years and older is expected to double, which means the need for caregiving is expected to increase with time.[18]

Caregiving can be a rewarding experience, but it can take a toll. Caregivers are at increased risk of illness and they often neglect their own health. Caregiving can have a physical and emotional impact on the caregiver.[18–21] It can lead to depression, anxiety, poor self-reported physical health, a compromised immune system, and an increase in the risk of early death.[18,20,21] Caregivers also commonly face financial strain caused by both the cost of health care as well as the impact caregiving has on the caregiver's work. Many caregivers report that their jobs have been affected by caregiving. These impacts include, but are not limited to, reducing the number of work hours and taking a leave of absence.[21]

The care of patients who require assistance depends on the health and abilities of the patient's caregivers. The needs of the caregivers must be considered. Clinicians can encourage the caregivers to have routine checkups with primary care physicians, use preventive services, have consistent health care coverage, and participate in self-care activities. Clinicians can help to connect caregivers with resources and support groups.[18] Connecting caregivers with other caregivers in similar situations can provide excellent social and emotional support. Caregivers often learn about more resources from each other.

Insurance Considerations

Patients with complex medical diagnoses commonly face significant financial burden in the United States. Medical services, procedures, and equipment are costly and the cost is not always covered by insurance. It is also common that insurances do not cover equipment or services for the purpose of reducing caregiver burden or reducing the caregiver's risk of injury. Patients and families often have to look for financial assistance elsewhere. Many fundraise and/or seek funding or grants from foundations that work to lessen this financial burden. Clinicians, case managers, and social workers can connect families with resources and help families navigate insurances as well.

When providing recommendations to families, it is also important to consider the cost-benefit analysis of the recommendation and make sure the family is aware of the cost of services to the best of the clinician's ability before providing a service or piece of equipment. Clinicians should also familiarize themselves with groups in their area that offer loaner and donated equipment. There are many groups that accept donated medical equipment to give to other patients in need for free. Some groups refurbish old equipment and even make patient-specific modifications to equipment that was donated to them and sell the equipment to patients at a reduced cost. This work is typically done in collaboration with the health care professionals that commonly work with that piece of equipment (eg, a physical therapist if the patient is trying to obtain a stander).

CLINICS CARE POINTS

- Patients with complex medical diagnoses should be followed by a multidisciplinary clinic. Multidisciplinary clinics allow improved patient outcomes[1,2] and reductions in patient mortality,[1,3] and can reduce health care costs.[2]

- Patient-centered and family-centered care allow better patient outcomes, improved patient and family satisfaction, more cost-effective care, improved staff satisfaction, and reductions in medical errors.[7]

- Laws exists that protect individuals with disabilities in the educational and work environments.

- Patients with disabilities should participate in regular physical activity. Physical activity has both physical and psychological benefits and can improve patients' quality of life.[16,17]

- Caregivers are at increased risk of illness and they often neglect their own health.[18–21] Caregiving can lead to depression, anxiety, poor self-reported physical health, a compromised immune system, and an increase in the risk of early death.[18,20,21]

DISCLOSURE

The author has nothing to disclose.

REFERENCES

1. Chen Y, Yang Y, Wang S, et al. Effectiveness of multidisciplinary care for chronic kidney disease in Taiwan: a 3-year prospective cohort study. Nephrol Dial Transplant 2013;28:671–82.
2. Joret M, Osman K, Dean A, et al. Multidisciplinary clinics reduce treatment costs and improve patient outcomes in diabetic foot disease. J Vasc Surg 2019;70: 806–14.

3. Wijeysundera H, Machado M, Wang X, et al. Cost-effectiveness of specialized multidisciplinary heart failure clinics in Ontario, Canada. Value Health 2010;13: 915–21.
4. Singh R, Kucukdeveci A, Grabljevec K, et al. The role of interdisciplinary teams in physical and rehabilitation medicine. J Rehabil Med 2018;50:673–8.
5. Hanson H, Harrington A, Nixon-Cave K. Implementing treatment frequency and duration guidelines in a hospital-based pediatric outpatient setting: administrative case report. Phys Ther 2015;95:678–84.
6. Bailes A, Reder R, Burch C. Development of guidelines for determining frequency of therapy services in a pediatric medical setting. Pediatr Phys Ther 2008;20: 194–8.
7. Policy statement: patient- and family-centered care and the pediatrician's role. Pediatrics 2012;129:394–404.
8. RESNA. Rehabilitation engineering and assistive technology society of North America 2020. Available at: resna.org. Accessed August 28, 2020.
9. Paleg G, Smith B, Glickman L. Systematic review and evidence-based clinical recommendations for dosing of pediatric supported standing programs. Pediatr Phys Ther 2013;25:232–47.
10. What is the Americans with Disabilities Act (ADA)?. Available at: adata.org/learn-about-ada. Accessed August 29, 2020.
11. Information and technical assistance on the Americans with disabilities act. 2020. Available at: Ada.gov. Accessed August 8, 2020.
12. The ADA: your employment rights as an individual with a disability. 2020. Available at: eeoc.gov. Accessed August 29, 2020.
13. Effgen S, Kaminker M. The educational environment. In: Palisano R, Orlin M, Schreiber J, editors. Campbell's physical therapy for children. Fifth Edition. St. Louis: Elsevier; 2017. p. 723–50.
14. IDEA. Individuals with disabilities education act. 2020. Available at: sites.ed.gov/idea/. Accessed August 28, 2020.
15. Woodmansee C, Hahne A, Imms C, et al. Comparing participation in physical recreation activities between children with disability and children with typical development: a secondary analysis of matched data. Res Dev Disabil 2016; 49-50:268–76.
16. Dubon M, Rovito C, Van Zandt DK, et al. Youth para and adaptive sports medicine. Curr Phys Med Rehabil Rep 2019;7:104–15.
17. Morris P. Physical activity recommendations for children and adolescents with chronic disease. Curr Sports Med Rep 2008;7:353–8.
18. Caregiving. Centers for disease control and prevention. 2019. Available at: cdc.gov. Accessed July 11, 2020.
19. Talley R, Crews J. Framing the public health of caregiving. Am J Public Health 2007;97:224–8.
20. Schulz R, Beach S. Caregiving as a risk factor for mortality: the caregiver health effects study. JAMA 1999;282:2215–9.
21. Caregiving in the United States 2020. AARP and National Alliance for Caregiving. Washington, DC: AARP; 2020

Medical Comorbidities and Complications Associated with Poliomyelitis and Its Sequelae

Lauren T. Shapiro, MD, MPH*, Andrew L. Sherman, MD, MS

KEYWORDS

- Poliomyelitis • Comorbidity • Cardiovascular deconditioning
- Postpoliomyelitis syndrome • Osteoporosis

KEY POINTS

- Persons living with sequelae of poliomyelitis often suffer from significant medical comorbidities negatively affecting their general health.
- Many of these comorbidities are in the cardiovascular realm and have a deleterious impact on the general health and functional level of polio survivors.
- Thus, we emphasize the need for early screening for these comorbid conditions, preventive interventions, and treatment to prevent their further decline when such conditions are identified.

INTRODUCTION

Widespread vaccination against polio has resulted in the elimination of new cases of paralytic poliomyelitis throughout most of the world. As of August 2020, wild poliovirus remains endemic in just 2 countries, Pakistan and Afghanistan.[1] Nevertheless, there remain significant numbers of individuals living with sequelae of poliomyelitis even in places that long ago saw their last new cases of infection, including the United States, where it has been eliminated for more than 30 years.[2] These sequelae include postpoliomyelitis syndrome (PPS), which affects between 25% and 40% of polio survivors. Those affected may develop worsening muscle weakness, fatigue, and/or joint pain many years following the initial infection.[3]

The authors have nothing to disclose.
Department of Physical Medicine and Rehabilitation, University of Miami Leonard M. Miller School of Medicine, PO Box 016960 (C-206), Miami, FL 33101, USA
* Corresponding author.
E-mail address: lxs973@med.miami.edu
Twitter: @ltshap (L.T.S.)

Phys Med Rehabil Clin N Am 32 (2021) 591–600
https://doi.org/10.1016/j.pmr.2021.02.010
1047-9651/21/© 2021 Elsevier Inc. All rights reserved.

Postpoliomyelitis syndrome, however, is far from the only cause of disability among polio survivors. Residual impairments, including weakness and gait dysfunction, are common and may elevate their risks for a number of conditions that in turn impact their overall health, quality of life, and function. Scoliosis, respiratory disorders, and mental health considerations are discussed in great detail in this issue.

The goal of this article was to provide a review of common comorbidities and sequelae found in those with a history of poliomyelitis, including those with and without PPS. We present the article in a problem-based format for the sake of organization. However, the reader must remember that many of these conditions occur together in our patients who must be looked at as the whole person that they are.

CARDIOVASCULAR CONDITIONS
Myocarditis

Myocarditis has been well-documented in the autopsy reports of some individuals who have died of poliomyelitis.[4–6] Moreover, electrocardiographic abnormalities are common in patients with poliomyelitis, usually appearing within the first 2 weeks of infection, suggesting myocarditis may be common in this population. The symptoms of myocardial involvement are nonspecific and little is known about the natural history of myocarditis in survivors of poliovirus infection.[7] Thus, a question that remains unanswered in the review of the literature is whether these findings of cardiac involvement during the acute phase of polio predispose those with late effects of polio to a higher incidence of heart disease. Viral myocarditis is often asymptomatic and may be self-limiting; however, some patients develop dilated cardiomyopathy and chronic heart failure.[8]

Deconditioning

Sequelae of poliomyelitis, such as weakness, musculoskeletal pain, and fatigue, may result in reduced physical activity and, accordingly, deconditioning. This, in turn, may increase the risk for cardiovascular diseases,[9] obesity, and other complications of immobility. Both those with and without PPS demonstrate reduced submaximal exercise capacity with incremental cycle ergometry tests when compared with healthy subjects.[10] Those with PPS exhibit a decline in aerobic capacity over a 3-year to 5-year period that is more rapid than is expected with aging.[11]

Cardiopulmonary endurance training is safe and effective for those with a history of poliomyelitis, although it is important to avoid muscle overuse. Improvement in maximal oxygen consumption has been observed in studies evaluating the effects of aerobic exercise programs on the fitness levels of individuals with poliomyelitis sequelae.[12,13] Additional benefits include perceived greater endurance and reduced fatigue during performance of their activities of daily living (ADLs) among program participants.[13] Kriz and colleagues[14] showed a significant improvement in persons with PPS who participated in a 16-week exercise program, 3 times a week, with each session lasting 20 minutes with upper limb cycle ergometry.

Ischemic Heart Disease

Survivors of poliomyelitis may be at increased risk for ischemic heart disease. Gawne and colleagues[15] performed a retrospective chart review of patients cared for in an outpatient post-polio clinic and found that more than 40% had more than 1 risk factor for coronary heart disease. A modestly increased risk for coronary artery disease has been observed among Danes with a history of poliomyelitis when compared with matched controls.[16] Ischemic heart disease is also more prevalent among Taiwanese survivors of paralytic poliomyelitis when compared with matched controls.[17] Signs and symptoms of heart disease, such as shortness of breath, leg edema, and fatigue, may be attributed to post-polio syndrome, resulting in a delay in diagnosis and treatment. As such, it is particularly important to screen this population for modifiable risk factors for heart disease and intervene when necessary.[15]

It is important to remember, however, when performing exercise stress testing, maximum exertion should be avoided in PPS due to the possibility of triggering "post-test fatigue." Activity should be prescribed based on submaximal tests. One example of a submaximal test is the 6-minute walk test. However, even that test can be problematic as, despite being a submaximal intensity test, patients with PPS often have biomechanical and orthopedic challenges that make the test impractical to perform.[18]

Dyslipidemia

Dyslipidemia is a highly prevalent comorbidity among individuals with a history of poliomyelitis. A retrospective chart review of patients cared for in an outpatient post-polio clinic in the United States revealed that more than half have hyperlipidemia (61.3%), making it more prevalent in this group than the general US population.[15] A cross-sectional study of post-polio patients in Sweden also found that hyperlipidemia was highly prevalent. Nevertheless, this study also found that it was less common among those with a history of poliomyelitis than their age-matched and gender-matched controls. They did, however, find that those in the post-polio group had lower levels of high density lipoproteins than the reference population.[19] Another study using data from Taiwan's National Health Insurance Research Database found a significantly higher prevalence of hyperlipidemia among survivors of paralytic poliomyelitis.[17] Agre and colleagues,[20] in a study of 64 post-polio patients, did find the prevalence to be much higher in men (66%) than women (25%). This retrospective study also found that only 19 patients of 50 identified with dyslipidemia had been given the diagnosis before the study and only 12 were receiving treatment. The study went on to conclude that their findings support the National Cholesterol Education Program's Adult Treatment Panel III statements that hypercholesterolemia is underdiagnosed and undertreated. Therefore, it is important to actively screen poliomyelitis survivors for lipid disorders and provide nutritional and exercise counseling and lipid-lowering medications when appropriate.[15]

Hypertension

Elevated blood pressure has been observed in acute poliomyelitis, and in some cases, it persists for months or years following infection.[21] Hypertension is also a very common comorbidity among polio survivors. It is the most common comorbid condition among polio survivors younger than 60 in Sweden.[22] In their retrospective chart review of patients cared for in an outpatient post-polio clinic, Gawne and colleagues[15] reported that half of the patients either had a history of hypertension or had elevated blood pressure. In their population-based study of poliomyelitis survivors in Taiwan, Kang and Lin[17] observed that hypertension was significantly more prevalent among these survivors than their matched controls. The need for hypertensive control in this population is paramount to avoid complications that may result in further disability.[7]

Peripheral Vascular Disease

Peripheral vascular disorders are also more prevalent among survivors of poliomyelitis. Nevertheless, their prevalence was less than 2% in the aforementioned study by Kang and Lin.[17] In addition to risks for atherosclerotic disease, those with limb paralysis may have loss of the muscle pump mechanism, which in turn may impede venous return to the heart.[23] This may result in chronic venous insufficiency and peripheral edema, for which compression therapy remains the recommended first-line treatment.[24]

OBESITY

Many of the preceding cardiovascular conditions also can be considered secondary consequences of obesity. However, most of the studies did conclude that independent of obesity and other risk factors, persons with polio were more likely than age-matched cohorts to have such conditions. But, there are conflicting data regarding whether a history of poliomyelitis elevates the risk for obesity. One might expect that one who is less mobile due to their chronic neurologic condition would be at an elevated risk for becoming obese.[25] Chang and colleagues[26] in a study of body composition in polio survivors did find an elevation in many concerning markers of obesity compared with controls matched by sex, age, body weight, and height. These markers included a 50% greater total body fat mass, significant increases in the regional fat mass in every part of the body, and a focal increase of fat mass in the thorax. Nearly all the subjects (94%) with poliomyelitis were obese according to standards of body composition. However, one-third of them had a body mass index (BMI) value of less than 25.0 kg/m^2. This confounding finding suggests that measures other than BMI should be used to decide if they are, in fact obese, and accordingly, at risk for many of the cardiovascular and neurologic risk factors that obese persons can suffer. The investigators suggest the possibility of creating a novel measure of BMI for polio survivors, as current BMI measures may significantly underestimate the prevalence of obesity in this population.

NEUROLOGIC CONDITIONS
Stroke

In a prospective, large population-based study of polio survivors in Taiwan, Wu and colleagues[27] found a prevalence of stroke that was more than 4 times that of age-matched and sex-matched controls. Moreover, they found that the prevalence of stroke among those who had both poliomyelitis and hypertension was more than 20%. A history of poliomyelitis was noted to be a significant risk factor for stroke in their cohort, independent of hypertension, diabetes mellitus, hyperlipidemia, and heart disease. Therefore, efforts to control blood pressure and promote an active lifestyle and normal body weight should be essential in the care of any post-polio patient and may reduce their elevated risk for stroke.

Dysphagia

Acute poliovirus infection may result in bulbar weakness, which in turn, may result in impairments in swallowing ability, speech, and the clearance of secretions.[28] Dysphagia is also seen in post-polio syndrome in survivors of both bulbar and non-bulbar forms of the disease.[29] Most affected patients report progressive symptoms and the use of compensatory strategies including head turning, tilting, and dietary modifications.[30] Videofluoroscopic swallow evaluations are recommended in the evaluation of post-polio patients with difficulty swallowing. Common findings include impaired tongue activity, unilateral transport of the bolus through the pharynx, and delayed esophageal motility.[29] Dysarthria and dysphonia are also common among individuals with dysphagia in the setting of post-polio syndrome.[30] Instruction in swallowing compensatory strategies is beneficial, as patients who comply with such strategies report fewer episodes of choking and feeling as though food is getting stuck while swallowing.[31]

Entrapment Neuropathy of the Upper Limbs

Upper limb entrapment neuropathies are very common among individuals with a history of poliomyelitis. Tsai and colleagues[32] reported a prevalence rate of 80% among their cohort of survivors of paralytic poliomyelitis in Taiwan. In their study, diagnosis was made with electrodiagnostic testing. Median mononeuropathy at the wrist was the most common entrapment neuropathy observed, and was present in more than 60% of their subjects. Ulnar neuropathies at the elbow and the wrist were also common. Risk factors for entrapment neuropathies among this group included being overweight or obese and the use of a cane, crutch, or wheelchair.[32,33]

Median mononeuropathy at the wrist (carpal tunnel syndrome [CTS]) can be particularly disabling in those with sequelae of poliomyelitis. The symptoms of hand numbness and weakness may limit their ability to ambulate (use their assistive devices), write, and/or work. CTS is often bilateral and, in those who use a single crutch or cane to ambulate, is more likely to develop on the side with which they hold their assistive device. Splints may help with the pain, numbness, and weakness they experience, but their use does not result in significant improvements with regard to ambulation or function. Carpal tunnel release surgery in the post-polio population similarly does not appear to significantly improve the function of those affected.[34]

Restless Legs Syndrome

Restless legs syndrome (RLS) is a common disorder among individuals with sequelae of poliomyelitis, including both those with and without PPS.[35] Having legs active at night can impair sleep significantly. Such deprivation may contribute to fatigue and impaired health-related quality of life in this population, although may respond well to treatment with dopamine agonist medications.[35,36]

Affected individuals have an urge to move the legs that is often, but not always, associated with an unpleasant sensation in the lower limbs. Patients typically describe a tingling or "creepy-crawly" sensation in their legs. Their symptoms are worse at night and during periods of inactivity and are at least partially relieved by movement.[37,38]

Although the pathophysiology of RLS in individuals with sequelae of poliomyelitis is not yet known, studies suggest an association between the 2 conditions. In a single-center study, Kumru and colleagues[35] reported more than 40% of those with polio sequelae met diagnostic criteria for RLS. Marin and colleagues[39] reported the prevalence of RLS in patients with PPS in their single-center study was 36%. Romigi and colleagues[36] found a significantly higher prevalence of RLS among people with PPS when compared with healthy controls. In a case series of patients with PPS and RLS, Marin and colleagues[38] reported a strong correlation between the age of onset of symptoms of both syndromes, with most patients reporting a concurrent onset.

BONE DISORDERS
Heterotopic Ossification

Heterotopic ossification (HO), the formation of bone in muscle and soft tissue, has been reported in survivors of paralytic poliomyelitis.[40,41] Affected individuals with HO may present with pain, edema, and restricted range of motion.[40] Those who have also sustained a traumatic injury, such as a fracture or dislocation, or who have undergone hip arthroplasty, may be at particularly high risk. Surgical resection may be necessary in cases in which the ectopic bone results in pain that cannot be controlled with conservative measures, significantly limits function, and/or puts the patient at risk for pressure sores. It is, however, recommended to delay surgery until the bone is fully matured, to reduce the risk of recurrence.[42]

Osteoporosis and Fractures

Osteoporosis and osteopenia are extremely prevalent among survivors of poliomyelitis, with Mohammed and colleagues[43] reporting rates of 56% and 40%, respectively. Postmenopausal women and middle-aged men are at particularly increased risk.[44] Smoking and reduced mobility are also important risk factors for osteoporosis in this population.[43] Among those with unilateral or asymmetrical lower limb weakness, the mean femoral bone density is significantly lower on the weaker side.[45] Patients with osteoporosis following poliomyelitis benefit from oral bisphosphonate therapy, which has been shown to improve their femoral neck bone mineral density as well as decrease their fracture risk.[46]

Fractures are common among poliomyelitis survivors and often occur secondary to falls. In a survey of polio survivors, Silver and Aiello[47] reported that 35% had experienced at least one bony fracture secondary to a fall. Adults with a history of polio have a significantly higher incidence of hip fractures when compared with matched controls.[48] More than 80% of femur fractures seen in this population are due to falls and most occur in the polio-affected limb. Despite the alarming rates of fractures, fewer than 25% were treated with anti-osteoporotic medications.[49] Of those with femur fractures requiring operative management, most do not return to their pre-injury walking capacity following surgery.[50]

Using a simple tool such as a dual energy X-ray absorptiometry (DEXA) scan on both the afflicted atrophic limb and the contralateral limb, as well as the lumbar spine for comparison, can help identify those who require treatment for reduced bone density. The DEXA scan of the femoral neck of the weaker limb of a patient with history of poliomyelitis, depicting a markedly reduced bone mineral density, is seen in **Fig. 1**. Treatment of osteoporosis and rehabilitation measures aimed at reducing the risk of falls are critical for preserving the functional status of aging poliomyelitis survivors.

PAIN DISORDERS

Long-standing pain is highly prevalent among survivors of poliomyelitis. Halstead and Rossi[51] reported on the results of a survey of more than 500 individuals with a history of poliomyelitis in which more than half of the respondents reported muscle and joint pain. Werhagen and Borg[52] reported that more than two-thirds of the patients cared for in a post-polio clinic in Stockholm had pain of at least 3 months' duration. They reported that most experienced nociceptive pain; those who reported neuropathic pain had other neurologic diagnoses to which the pain was attributed.

It is important to note that post-polio syndrome and fibromyalgia have overlapping symptoms, namely chronic diffuse pain and fatigue. Interestingly, Trojan and Cashman[53] found that more than 10% of patients cared for in a post-polio clinic met clinical criteria for the diagnosis of fibromyalgia. Approximately half of the patients in their case series had improvement in pain with low-dose amitriptyline given at night.

PREGNANCY AND PERINATAL OUTCOMES

Poliovirus infection and its sequelae may greatly impact the course and outcome of an affected woman's pregnancy. Before widespread immunization, maternal infection late in pregnancy was associated with transplacental transmission of the virus, with

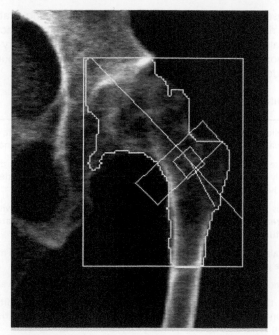

Fig. 1. The DEXA scan of the femoral neck of a postmenopausal woman with a remote history of poliomyelitis with residual left lower limb weakness (Bone mineral density: 0.271 g/cm^2, T-score: −5.2).

rare reports of newborn paralysis. Polio infection was also associated with increased rates of spontaneous abortions and stillbirths.[54]

Pregnancy in survivors of poliomyelitis is also associated with an increased risk for complications and adverse perinatal outcomes. A cohort study using data from the national birth registry in Norway revealed that polio survivors are more likely to have deliveries complicated by obstruction of the birth process and have cesarean deliveries at a higher rate than other mothers (13.2% vs 8.3%). The infants of mothers who had poliomyelitis had a lower mean birth weight. The risk of perinatal death was also increased in this group, at slightly more than 2%. Pregnant women with a history of poliomyelitis were also noted to have higher rates of preeclampsia, vaginal bleeding, and urinary tract infections.[55] There are concerns that pregnancy may be particularly hazardous for women with chronic respiratory failure due to poliomyelitis. Nevertheless, successful pregnancies among such women dependent on noninvasive intermittent positive pressure ventilation have been reported.[56]

SUMMARY

Although poliovirus is no longer endemic through most of the world, many are still living with sequelae of their remote infections. Moreover, survivors of poliomyelitis often have comorbid conditions that may impact their overall health, comfort, mobility, ability to perform their ADLs, and, potentially, pregnancy and perinatal outcomes. Screening for and the treatment of hypertension, dyslipidemia, and reduced bone density among this population is critically important. Rehabilitation measures, including cardiopulmonary exercise training, fall prevention education, and the instruction of those with dysphagia in compensatory swallowing strategies, may also help mitigate the risk of complications, including deconditioning, fractures, and aspiration. Chronic pain is also very prevalent among those with a history of poliomyelitis, including both those with and without PPS. Identification of the sources of pain are necessary to guide the optimal individualized treatment strategy.

CLINICS CARE POINTS

- Sequelae of poliomyelitis may result in reduced mobility and, as a result, deconditioning, which in turn may increase the risk for cardiovascular diseases, obesity, and falls.

- Many of these sequelae are in the cardiovascular realm, as hypertension, dyslipidemia, and stroke are highly prevalent among survivors of poliomyelitis and have a deleterious impact on the general health and function of this population.

- As osteoporosis and osteopenia are also common among those with a history of poliomyelitis, treatment with bisphosphonates and fall risk reduction strategies are crucial to prevent fractures.

- Chronic pain is also highly prevalent among survivors of poliomyelitis and may be secondary to degenerative joint disease, scoliosis, and/or entrapment neuropathies.

- Fibromyalgia and RLS are also common in this population and respond well to treatment.

- We emphasize the need for early screening for these comorbid conditions, preventive interventions, and control of the modifiable risk factors to minimize the risk of further disability among survivors of poliomyelitis.

REFERENCES

1. Polio vaccines: WHO position paper – March, 2016, week. Epidemiol Rec 2016; 91(12):145–68.
2. Polio elimination in the U.S. Centers for Disease Control and Prevention. 2019. Available at: https://www.cdc.gov/polio/what-is-polio/polio-us.html. Accessed August 29, 2020.
3. Post-polio syndrome. Centers for Disease Control and Prevention. 2019. Available at: https://www.cdc.gov/polio/what-is-polio/pps.html. Accessed August 29, 2020.
4. Ludden TE, Edwards JE. Carditis in poliomyelitis; an anatomic study of 35 cases and review of the literature. Am J Pathol 1949;25(3):357–81.
5. Spain DM, Bradess VA, Parsonnet V. Myocarditis in poliomyelitis. Am Heart J 1950;40(3):336–44.
6. Galpine JF, Wilson WC. Occurrence of myocarditis in paralytic poliomyelitis. Br Med J 1959;2(5163):1379–81.
7. Weinstein L. Cardiovascular disturbances in poliomyelitis. Circulation 1957;15(5): 735–56.
8. Kearney MT, Cotton JM, Richardson PJ, et al. Viral myocarditis and dilated cardiomyopathy: mechanisms, manifestations, and management. Postgrad Med J 2001;77(903):4–10.
9. Orsini M, Lopes AJ, Guimarães FS, et al. Currents issues in cardiorespiratory care of patients with post-polio syndrome. Arq Neuropsiquiatr 2016;74(7):574–9.
10. Nollet F, Beelen A, Sargeant AJ, et al. Submaximal exercise capacity and maximal power output in polio subjects. Arch Phys Med Rehabil 2001;82(12): 1678–85.
11. Stanghelle JK, Festvåg LV. Postpolio syndrome: a 5 year follow-up. Spinal Cord 1997;35(8):503–8.

12. Dean E, Ross J. Movement energetics of individuals with a history of poliomyelitis. Arch Phys Med Rehabil 1993;74(5):478–83.

13. Jones DR, Speier J, Canine K, et al. Cardiorespiratory responses to aerobic training by patients with postpoliomyelitis sequelae. JAMA 1989;261(22):3255–8.

14. Kriz JL, Jones DR, Speier JL, et al. Cardiorespiratory responses to upper extremity aerobic training by postpolio subjects. Arch Phys Med Rehabil 1992;73(1):49–54.

15. Gawne AC, Wells KR, Wilson KS. Cardiac risk factors in polio survivors. Arch Phys Med Rehabil 2003;84(5):694–6.

16. Nielsen NM, Rostgaard K, Askgaard D, et al. Life-long morbidity among Danes with poliomyelitis. Arch Phys Med Rehabil 2004;85(3):385–91.

17. Kang JH, Lin HC. Comorbidity profile of poliomyelitis survivors in a Chinese population: a population-based study. J Neurol 2011;258(6):1026–33.

18. Vreede KS, Henriksson J, Borg K, et al. Gait characteristics and influence of fatigue during the 6-minute walk test in patients with post-polio syndrome. J Rehabil Med 2013;45(9):924–8.

19. Melin E, Kahan T, Borg K. Elevated blood lipids are uncommon in patients with post-polio syndrome–a cross sectional study. BMC Neurol 2015;15:67.

20. Agre JC, Rodriguez AA, Sperling KB. Plasma lipid and lipid concentrations in symptomatic post-polio patients. Arch Phys Med Rehabil 1990;71:393–4.

21. Ostfeld AM. Sustained hypertension after poliomyelitis. Arch Intern Med 1961; 107:551–7.

22. Werhagen L, Borg K. Survey of young patients with polio and a foreign background at a Swedish post-polio outpatient clinic. Neurol Sci 2016;37(10): 1597–601.

23. Frustace SJ. Poliomyelitis: late and unusual sequelae. Am J Phys Med 1987; 66(6):328–37.

24. Eberhardt RT, Raffetto JD. Chronic venous insufficiency. Circulation 2014;130(4): 333–46.

25. Fitzmaurice C, Kanarek N, Fitzgerald S. Primary prevention among working age USA adults with and without disabilities. Disabil Rehabil 2011;33:343–51.

26. Chang KH, Lai CH, Chen SC, et al. Body composition assessment in Taiwanese individuals with poliomyelitis. Arch Phys Med Rehabil 2011;92:1092–7.

27. Wu CH, Liou TH, Chen HH, et al. Stroke risk in poliomyelitis survivors: a nationwide population-based study. Arch Phys Med Rehabil 2012;93(12):2184–8.

28. Cohen JI. Enterovirus, parechovirus, and reovirus infections. In: Jameson J, Fauci AS, Kasper DL, et al, editors. Harrison's principles of internal medicine, 2018. New York: McGraw-Hill. Available at: https://accessmedicine-mhmedical-com. access.library.miami.edu/content.aspx?bookid=2129&sectionid=192025777. Accessed August 16, 2020.

29. Sonies BC, Dalakas MC. Dysphagia in patients with the post-polio syndrome. N Engl J Med 1991;324(17):1162–7.

30. Buchholz D, Jones B. Dysphagia occurring after polio. Dysphagia 1991;6(3): 165–9.

31. Silbergleit AK, Waring WP, Sullivan MJ, et al. Evaluation, treatment, and follow-up results of post polio patients with dysphagia. Otolaryngol Head Neck Surg 1991; 104(3):333–8.

32. Tsai HC, Hung TH, Chen CC, et al. Prevalence and risk factors for upper extremity entrapment neuropathies in polio survivors. J Rehabil Med 2009;41(1):26–31.

33. Werner R, Waring W, Davidoff G. Risk factors for median mononeuropathy of the wrist in postpoliomyelitis patients. Arch Phys Med Rehabil 1989;70(6):464–7.

34. Waring WP 3rd, Werner RA. Clinical management of carpal tunnel syndrome in patients with long-term sequelae of poliomyelitis. J Hand Surg Am 1989;14(5):865–9.
35. Kumru H, Portell E, Barrio M, et al. Restless legs syndrome in patients with sequelae of poliomyelitis. Parkinsonism Relat Disord 2014;20(10):1056–8.
36. Romigi A, Pierantozzi M, Placidi F, et al. Restless legs syndrome and post polio syndrome: a case-control study. Eur J Neurol 2015;22(3):472–8.
37. Allen RP, Picchietti DL, Garcia-Borreguero D, et al. Restless legs syndrome/Willis-Ekbom disease diagnostic criteria: updated International Restless Legs Syndrome Study Group (IRLSSG) consensus criteria–history, rationale, description, and significance. Sleep Med 2014;15(8):860–73.
38. Marin LF, Carvalho LB, Prado LB, et al. Restless legs syndrome in post-polio syndrome: a series of 10 patients with demographic, clinical and laboratorial findings. Parkinsonism Relat Disord 2011;17(7):563–4.
39. Marin LF, Carvalho LBC, Prado LBF, et al. Restless legs syndrome is highly prevalent in patients with post-polio syndrome. Sleep Med 2017;37:147–50.
40. Costello FV, Brown A. Myositis ossificans complicating anterior poliomyelitis. J Bone Joint Surg Br 1951;33-B(4):594–7.
41. Hess WE. Myositis ossificans occurring in poliomyelitis; report of a case. AMA Arch Neurol Psychiatry 1951;66(5):606–9.
42. Meyers C, Lisiecki J, Miller S, et al. Heterotopic ossification: a comprehensive review. JBMR Plus 2019;3(4):e10172.
43. Mohammad AF, Khan KA, Galvin L, et al. High incidence of osteoporosis and fractures in an aging post-polio population. Eur Neurol 2009;62(6):369–74.
44. Haziza M, Kremer R, Benedetti A, et al. Osteoporosis in a postpolio clinic population. Arch Phys Med Rehabil 2007;88(8):1030–5.
45. Grill B, Levangie PK, Cole M, et al. Bone mineral density among individuals with residual lower limb weakness after Polio. PM R 2019;11(5):470–5.
46. Alvarez A, Kremer R, Weiss DR, et al. Response of postpoliomyelitis patients to bisphosphonate treatment. PM R 2010;2(12):1094–103.
47. Silver JK, Aiello DD. Polio survivors: falls and subsequent injuries. Am J Phys Med Rehabil 2002;81(8):567–70.
48. Wu CH, Huang SW, Lin YN, et al. Adults with polio are at risk of hip fracture from middle age: a nationwide population-based cohort study. Injury 2019;50(3):738–43.
49. Goerss J, Atkinson E, Windeback A, et al. Fractures in aging population of poliomyelitis survivors: a community based study in Olmsted County, Minnesota. Mayo Clin Proc 1994;69:333–9.
50. Gellman YN, Khoury A, Liebergall M, et al. Outcome of femoral fractures in poliomyelitis patients. Int Orthop 2019;43(11):2607–12.
51. Halstead LS, Rossi CD. New problems in old polio patients: results of a survey of 539 polio survivors. Orthopedics 1985;8(7):845–50.
52. Werhagen L, Borg K. Analysis of long-standing nociceptive and neuropathic pain in patients with post-polio syndrome. J Neurol 2010;257(6):1027–31.
53. Trojan DA, Cashman NR. Fibromyalgia is common in a postpoliomyelitis clinic. Arch Neurol 1995;52(6):620–4.
54. Ornoy A, Tenenbaum A. Pregnancy outcome following infections by coxsackie, echo, measles, mumps, hepatitis, polio and encephalitis viruses. Reprod Toxicol 2006;21(4):446–57.
55. Veiby G, Daltveit AK, Gilhus NE. Pregnancy, delivery and perinatal outcome in female survivors of polio. J Neurol Sci 2007;258(1–2):27–32.
56. Bach JR. Successful pregnancies for ventilator users. Am J Phys Med Rehabil 2003;82(3):226–9.

Moving?

Make sure your subscription moves with you!

To notify us of your new address, find your **Clinics Account Number** (located on your mailing label above your name), and contact customer service at:

Email: journalscustomerservice-usa@elsevier.com

800-654-2452 (subscribers in the U.S. & Canada)
314-447-8871 (subscribers outside of the U.S. & Canada)

Fax number: 314-447-8029

Elsevier Health Sciences Division
Subscription Customer Service
3251 Riverport Lane
Maryland Heights, MO 63043

*To ensure uninterrupted delivery of your subscription, please notify us at least 4 weeks in advance of move.

Printed and bound by CPI Group (UK) Ltd, Croydon, CR0 4YY

03/10/2024

01040484-0014